Sirtfood Diet Cookbook

Over 100 Easy and Delicious Recipes to Burn Fat, Lose Weight, Get Lean and Feel Great!

Dr I. Pot

COPYRIGHT

CONTENTS

INTRODUCTION

To start the diet, members are required to follow a fourteen day plan which incorporates diminishing your calorie consumption and devouring 'Sirtfood green juices'.

"For the main week you confine your [calorie] admission to 1000 calories which incorporates expending three sirtfood green juices and one sirtfood-rich dinner daily," Michele shares.

"The next week you up your admission to 1500 calories every day and devour two sirtfood-rich dinners and two green juices."

Long haul there is no specific diet, yet an eating plan high in sirtfoods is supported alongside joining the diet's mark green juices.

The diet's makers guarantee the diet will prompt fast weight loss while keeping up muscle and mass and shielding you from incessant illness.

When Grammy Award-winning vocalist Adele uncovered her unbelievable 40kg weight loss toward the start of the year, those prepared to invite 2020 with new health and wellness objectives were anxious to discover exactly what her mystery was.

Alongside a recently discovered love for Reformer Pilates, the 31-year-old likewise followed a Sirtfood eating plan, and when we found it remembered chocolate and red wine for its rundown of 'affirmed' foods, we'd lie if we said it didn't provoke our curiosity.

While the keto diet re-wired what number of us think about fat with its high-fat eating plan that increased a faction following with its quick weight loss claims, could the Sirtfood diet change how we feel about regular 'treat' foods like red wine and chocolate?

Michele says it's nothing unexpected that individuals may see fast weight loss if they're confining their calorie consumption, especially during that first seven day stretch of the diet, however says she's extremely careful about urging individuals to tally calories.

She does, notwithstanding, see a colossal advantage in expanding your admission of sirtuin-rich foods, saying any diet rich in whole foods without included sugars will be gainful for your health.

She includes, "Sirtfoods actuate fat consuming, yet additionally advance muscle development, support and fix. Eating food normally rich in sirtuin activators might be healthier, progressively viable – and less expensive – option to polyphenol supplements."

So there you have it. While the Sirtfood diet has the correct thought in empowering the expansion of entire foods we ought to devour, its consolation of calorie tallying isn't really the healthiest methodology you could take when it goes to your wellbeing venture.

Concentrating on eating a balanced, sirtfood-rich diet and consolidating ordinary development into your day is consistently an extraordinary advance towards a fitter, healthier you.

CHAPTER 1: WHAT IS THE SIRT DIET

Propelled initially in 2016, the Sirtfood diet stays an intriguing issue and includes supporters embracing a diet rich in 'sirtfoods'. As indicated by the diet's authors, these exceptional foods work by enacting specific proteins in the body called sirtuins. Sirtuins are accepted to shield cells in the body from passing on when they are under pressure and are thought to direct irritation, digestion and the maturing procedure. It's idea that sirtuins impact the body's capacity to consume fat and lift digestion, bringing about a seven pound weight loss seven days while looking after muscle. In any case, a few specialists accept this is probably not going to be exclusively fat loss, however will rather reflect changes in glycogen stores from skeletal muscle and the liver.

The diet

So what are these otherworldly 'sirtfoods'? The ten most basic include:

- Green tea
- Dull chocolate (that is in any event 85 percent cocoa)

- Apples
- Citrus natural products
- Parsley
- Turmeric
- Kale
- Blueberries
- Tricks
- Red wine

The diet is separated into two stages; the underlying stage keeps going multi week and includes limiting calories to 1000kcal for three days, expending three sirtfood green juices and one supper rich in sirtfoods every day. The juices incorporate kale, celery, rocket, parsley, green tea and lemon. Dinners incorporate turkey escalope with sage, escapades and parsley, chicken and kale curry and prawn pan sear with buckwheat noodles. From days four to seven, vitality admissions are expanded to 1500kcal including two sirtfood green juices and two sirtfood-rich suppers daily.

In spite of the fact that the diet advances healthy foods, it's prohibitive in both your food decisions and every day calories, particularly during the underlying stages. It additionally includes drinking juice, with the sums proposed during stage one surpassing the present every day rules.

The subsequent stage is known as the upkeep stage which keeps going 14 days where consistent weight loss happens. The creators trust it's an economical and sensible approach to get in shape. In any case, concentrating on weight loss isn't what the diet is about – it's intended to be tied in with eating the best foods nature brings to the table. Long haul they suggest eating three balanced sirtfood rich suppers daily alongside one sirtfood green juice.

Dietitian Emer Delaney says:

'From the outset, this isn't a diet I would prompt for my customers. Planning to have 1000kcal for three back to back days is amazingly difficult and I accept most of individuals would be not able to accomplish it. Taking a gander at the rundown of foods, you can see they are the kind of things that often show up on a 'healthy food list', anyway it is smarter to support these as a major aspect of a healthy balanced diet. Having a glass of red wine or a modest quantity of chocolate every so often won't do us any mischief - I wouldn't suggest them consistently. We ought to likewise be eating a blend of different foods grown from the ground and not only those on the rundown.

'As far as weight loss and boosting digestion, individuals may have encountered a seven pound weight loss on the scales, however as far as I can tell this will be liquid. Consuming and losing fat requires some serious energy so it is amazingly improbable this weight loss is a loss of fat. I would be extremely careful of any diet that suggests quick and unexpected weight loss as this basically isn't feasible and will more than likely be a loss of liquid. When individuals come back to their ordinary dietary patterns, they will recapture the weight. Gradual weight loss is the key and for this we have to confine calories and increment our action levels. Gobbling balanced customary suppers comprised of low GI foods, lean protein, products of the soil and keeping all around hydrated is the most secure approach to get in shape.

At its center, the way to getting more fit is truly basic: Create a calorie shortage either by expanding your calorie consume exercises or diminishing your caloric admission. Be that as it may, imagine a scenario in which you could avoid the dieting and rather initiate a "thin quality" without the requirement for serious calorie limitation. This is the reason of The Sirtfood Diet, composed by nourishment specialists Aidan Goggins and Glen Matten. The best approach to do it, they contend, is sirtfoods.

Sirtfoods are wealthy in supplements that initiate a purported "thin quality" called sirtuin. As per Goggins and Matten, the "thin quality" is initiated when a deficiency of vitality is made after you limit calories. Sirtuins got fascinating to the sustenance world in 2003 when specialists found that resveratrol, a compound found in red wine, had a similar impact on life range as calorie limitation however it was accomplished without diminishing admission. (Discover the authoritative truth about wine and its health benefits.)

In the 2015 pilot study (directed by Goggins and Matten) testing the adequacy of sirtuins, the 39 members lost a normal of seven pounds in seven days. Those outcomes sound great; however it's imperative to understand this is a little example size concentrated over a brief timeframe. Weight-loss specialists additionally have their questions about the elevated guarantees. "The cases made are theoretical and

14

extrapolate from considers which were for the most part centered on straightforward living beings (like yeast) at the cell level. What occurs at the cell level doesn't really mean what occurs in the human body at the full scale level," says Adrienne Youdim, M.D., the chief of the Center for Weight Loss and Nutrition in Beverly Hills, CA. (Here, look at the best and most noticeably terrible diets to follow this year.)

What foods are high in sirtuins?

The book contains a rundown of the main 20 foods that are high in sirtuins, which sounds more like a slanting food list than another, advanced diet. Models include: arugula, chilies, espresso, green tea, Medjool dates, red wine, turmeric, pecans, and the health-cognizant top choice kale. Dr. Youdim takes note of that while the foods being advanced are healthy, they won't really advance weight loss all alone.

What does the diet involve?

The diet is executed in two stages. Stage one keeps going three days and limits calories to 1,000 every day, comprising of three green juices and one sirtfood-endorsed dinner. Stage two endures four days and raises the day by day allocation to 1,500 calories for each day with two green juices and two suppers.

After these stages, there is a support plan that isn't centered around calories yet rather on reasonable bits, even dinners, and topping off on essentially sirtfoods. The 14-day upkeep plan highlights three suppers, one green juice, and a couple sirtfood chomp snacks. Adherents are likewise urged to finish 30 minutes of action five days per week-per government proposals however it isn't the primary focal point of the arrangement.

What are the advantages?

You will get in shape if you follow this diet intently. "Regardless of whether you're eating 1,000 calories of tacos, 1,000 calories of kale, or 1,000 calories of snicker doodles, you will get more fit at 1,000 calories!" says Dr. Youdim. However, she additionally calls attention to that you can have accomplishment with a progressively sensible calorie limitation. The commonplace every day caloric admission of somebody not on a careful nutritional plan is 2,000 to 2,200, so diminishing to 1,500 is as yet limiting and would be a successful weight-loss methodology for most, she says.

Are there any safeguards?

This arrangement is severe with little squirm room or replacements, and weight loss must be kept up if the low caloric admission is likewise kept up, making it difficult to hold fast to long haul. That implies any weight you lost in the initial seven days is probably going to be restored after you finish, says Dr. Youdin. Her fundamental concern? "Constraining protein admission with juices will bring about a loss of bulk. Losing muscle is equal with dropping your metabolic rate or 'digestion,' making weight upkeep progressively difficult," she says.

Last Thoughts

By and large, Dr. Youdim would not suggest this diet. There are different ways that you can decrease calorie consumption without being so prohibitive in the foods that you eat. All things considered, the diet isn't really "unhealthy" so she wouldn't really alert against it if a patient discovered achievement.

If you do follow this arrangement, make certain to eat a lot of protein and fluctuate the foods you eat to forestall nutrient insufficiencies. Our take? The diet is fantastically severe and its viability has not been satisfactorily demonstrated. You're greatly improved off building up a lifestyle of eating an assortment of entire foods in the extents that suit your individual needs.

How It Works

Celeb gets in shape. Celeb gets shot appearing to be unique. Fans go wild and are *dying* to know precisely how they did it. Enter: Adele! The artist was spotted a year ago (and again on an ongoing get-away in Anguilla) with a recognizably slimmer figure, and individuals are overly inquisitive about the eating plan she supposedly follows: the Sirtfood Diet.

While Adele hasn't spoken openly about her weight loss, the New York Post guaranteed that she has shed 50 pounds by following the eating plan (and her name was initially appended to the diet in 2016). A previous mentor of the star additionally as of late revealed to The Sun that she accepts the adjustments in Adele's physical make-up boil down to "90 percent diet."

The Sirtfood Diet has purportedly gotten love from various celebs notwithstanding the "Somebody Like You" artist, including Pippa Middleton and popular competitors like previous professional fighter David Haye.

The short form: The Sirtfood Diet is supposed to be wealthy in foods that contain a specific supplement that helps trigger qualities in the body associated with fat loss and fat stockpiling (more on this in a moment). Furthermore, a few people say they love it because there are some truly tasty foods that have these exceptional supplements (greetings, wine and chocolate), so you don't feel denied.

The Sirtfood Diet

But...is the Sirtfood Diet unrealistic? Here's all that you have to think about the gracious so-buzzy-right-now weight-loss strategy, with contribution from sustenance specialists Caroline Apovian, MD, chief of the Nutrition and Weight Management Center at the Boston Medical Center, and Edwina Clark, RD, head of nourishment and health for Yummly.

To begin with, what is the Sirtfood Diet precisely?

The diet originates from the book of a similar name. The creators—Aidan Goggins and Glen Matten—of The Sirtfood Diet exhort eating for the most part foods rich in sirtuins, a kind of protein in plant foods. "The eating plan itself is intended to 'turn on' the sirtuin qualities (especially SIRT-1), which are accepted to support digestion, increment fat consuming, battle aggravation, and check hunger," says Clark.

Early examinations propose that calorie limitation and resveratrol (a polyphenol found in foods like grapes, blueberries, and peanuts), initiate the SIRT-1 quality, and these two standards support the Sirtfood way to deal with eating.

What does the arrangement involve?

The diet endures a sum of three weeks and is isolated into two stages.

Stage one: You restrain yourself to three Sirtfood green juices (containing kale, arugula, parsley, celery, green apple, lemon squeeze, and green tea) and one Sirtfood-rich dinner every day, totaling around 1,000 calories every day, says Dr. Apovian, MD. For the following four days, you drink two Sirtfood green squeezes and eat two Sirtfood-rich suppers, which brings your calorie aggregate to around 1,500 every day.

Stage two: This is the support stage, which keeps going 14 days. During those fourteen days, you should have three Sirtfood-rich dinners and one Sirtfood green squeeze day by day.

When those three weeks are up, there's no set intend to follow. To proceed on the Sirtfood way, you should simply change every one of your suppers to incorporate whatever number Sirtfoods as would be prudent. Exercise is likewise empowered (30 minutes of action, five days per week), however getting sweat-soaked isn't the fundamental focal point of the weight-loss plan.

Sooo, would you be able to get more fit on the diet?

The Sirtfood Diet incorporates numerous nutritious foods that are gainful for weight loss, for example, celery, kale, green tea, Medjool dates, lean chicken, lean red meat, and parsley, says Dr. Apovian. The diet likewise confines or kills numerous foods that are known to cause weight increase, for example, refined flours, included sugars, and prepared foods with almost no dietary benefit. Also, because of that incredibly low calorie admission, devotees will probably shed pounds gave they stay on track, she says.

"Proof to date recommends that caloric limitation and discontinuous fasting can be a successful technique for weight loss and improving metabolic health," says Clark. "Be that as it may, this may not be proper for everybody," she says.

Are there any drawbacks?

The drawn out manageability of this arrangement is sketchy. When you're past the initial not many weeks, there's no eating technique to follow other than adding more Sirtfoods to every dinner. This makes the diet significantly more adaptable than most, which is an immense advantage, yet a three-week extended length of hardship could without much of a stretch lead to gorging during stage two, eventually putting you back at the starting point.

Regardless of whether you're uber-restrained, this is as yet an intense diet to follow. "An insignificant 1,000 calories will leave the vast majority feeling extremely eager," says Dr. Apovian. Also, if you're not an aficionado of green squeeze, a staple of the main week, that will make you considerably hungrier, she says. Likewise, since the majority of the weight loss in stage one is water weight, it will return directly on once you continue typical eating, she says.

In addition, following any diet that does exclude a healthy measure of protein (e.g., during the main seven day stretch of the Sirtfood Diet), may bring about muscle loss and a more slow digestion, says Dr. Apovian. To get in shape and keep it off, building muscle through eating a lot of protein and working out with weights is principal.

On all that, look into on SIRT-1 initiating foods is still particularly in its outset, so it's hazy in the case of devouring polyphenol-rich foods substantially affects weight in everybody. "Weight is a multi-faceted idea, including complex associations between our one of kind hereditary cosmetics and our diet, development designs, rest propensities, and passionate state," notes Clark.

At last, eating a diet wealthy in an assortment of healthy foods, including lean protein sources, different leafy foods, and entire grains is a healthier, increasingly practical approach to get thinner and keep it off, says Dr. Apovian.

The Power of Sirtuins

Sirtuins help control your cell health. This is what you have to think about how they work, what they can accomplish for your body, and why they depend on NAD+ to work.

Sirtuins are a group of proteins that direct cell health. Sirtuins assume a key job in controlling cell homeostasis. Homeostasis includes keeping the cell in balance. Be that as it may, sirtuins can just capacity within the sight of NAD+, nicotinamide adenine dinucleotide, a coenzyme found in every single living cell.

How Sirtuins Regulate Cellular Health with NAD+

Think about your body's cells like an office. In the workplace, there are numerous individuals chipping away at different errands with an extreme objective:

remain gainful and satisfy the crucial the organization in a proficient way for whatever length of time that conceivable. In the cells, there are numerous pieces taking a shot at different assignments with an extreme objective, as well: remain healthy and work effectively for whatever length of time that conceivable. Similarly as needs in the organization change, because of different inward and outer components, so do needs in the cells. Somebody needs to run the workplace, controlling what completes when, who will do it and when to switch course. In the workplace, that would be your CEO. In the body, at the cell level, it's your sirtuins.

Sirtuins are a group of seven proteins that assume a job in cell health. Sirtuins can just capacity within the sight of NAD+, nicotinamide adenine dinucleotide, a coenzyme found in every single living cell. NAD+ is fundamental to cell digestion and several other organic procedures. If sirtuins are an organization's CEO, then NAD+ is the cash that pays the compensation of the CEO and workers, all while keeping the lights on and the workplace space lease paid. An organization, and the body, can't work without it. Be that as it may, levels of NAD+ decay with age, restricting the capacity of sirtuins with age also. Like everything in the human body, it isn't so straightforward. Sirtuins oversee everything that occurs in your cells.

Sirtuins Are Proteins. I'm not catching that's meaning?

Sirtuins are a group of proteins. Protein may seem like dietary protein — what's found in beans and meats and well, protein shakes — yet for this situation we're discussing eBooks called proteins, which work all through the body's phones in various different capacities. Consider proteins the divisions at an organization, every one concentrating on its own specific capacity while planning with different offices.

A notable protein in the body is hemoglobin, which is a piece of the globin group of proteins and is liable for shipping oxygen all through your blood. The myoglobin is the hemoglobin's partner, and together they make up the globin family.

Your body has almost 60,000 groups of proteins — a ton of offices! — and sirtuins are one of those families. While hemoglobin is one out of a group of two proteins, sirtuins are a group of seven.

Of the seven sirtuins in the cell, three of them work in the mitochondria, three of them work in the core and one of them works in the cytoplasm, each assuming an assortment of jobs. The fundamental job of sirtuins, in any case, is that they expel acetyl bunches from different proteins.

Acetyl bunches control specific responses. They're physical labels on proteins that different proteins perceive will respond with them. If proteins are the branches of the cell and DNA is the CEO, the acetyl bunches are the accessibility status of every office head. For instance, if a protein is accessible then the sirtuin can work with it to get something going, similarly as the CEO can work with an accessible office head to get something going.

Sirtuins work with acetyl bunches by doing what's called deacetylation. This implies they perceive there's an acetyl bunch on an atom then expel the acetyl gathering, which tees up the pbook for its activity. One way that sirtuins work is by evacuating acetyl gatherings (deacetylating) natural proteins, for example, histones. For instance, sirtuins deacetylate histones, proteins that are a piece of a dense type of

DNA called chromatin. The histone is an enormous cumbersome protein that the DNA folds itself over. Consider it a Christmas tree, and the DNA strand is the strand of lights. When the histones have an acetyl gathering, the chromatin is open, or loosened up.

This loosened up chromatin implies the DNA is being translated, a basic procedure. In any case, it doesn't have to remain loosened up, as it's helpless against harm in this position, practically like the Christmas lights could get tangled or the bulbs can get harmed when they're clumsy or up for a really long time. When the histones are deacetylated by sirtuins, the chromatin is shut, or firmly and perfectly twisted, which means quality articulation is halted, or hushed.

We've just thought about sirtuins for around 20 years, and their essential capacity was found during the 1990s. From that point forward, analysts have run to examine them, identifying their significance while likewise bringing up issues about what else we can find out about them.

The Discovery and History of Sirtuins

Geneticist Dr. Amar Klar found the first sirtuin, called SIR2, during the 1970s, identifying it as a quality that controlled the capacity of yeast cells to mate. A long time later, during the 1990s, specialists discovered different qualities that were homologous — comparative in structure — to SIR2 in different creatures like worms, natural product flies, and these SIR2 homologues were then named sirtuins. There were different quantities of sirtuins in every creature. For instance, yeast has five sirtuins, microscopic organisms has one, mice have seven, and people have seven.

The way that sirtuins were found across species implies they were "rationed" with development. Qualities that are "moderated" have widespread capacities in numerous or all species. What was at this point to be known, however, was the means by which significant sirtuins would end up being.

In 1991, Elysium fellow benefactor and MIT scientist Leonard Guarente, nearby alumni understudies Nick Austriaco and Brian Kennedy, led analyses to more readily see how yeast matured. By some coincidence,

Austriaco attempted to develop societies of different yeast strains from tests he had put away in his cooler for a considerable length of time, which made an upsetting domain for the strains. Just a portion of these strains could develop from here, however Guarente and his group identified an example: The strains of yeast that endure the best in the refrigerator were additionally the longest lived. This gave direction to Guarente so he could concentrate exclusively on these long-living strains of yeast.

This prompted the identification of SIR2 as a quality that advanced life span in yeast. It's imperative to take note of that to date there isn't yet proof that this examination can be extrapolated to people and more research is required on SIR2's belongings in people. The Guarente lab subsequently found that expelling SIR2 abbreviated yeast life length significantly, while in particular, expanding the quantity of duplicates of the SIR2 quality from one to two expanded the life range in yeast. Yet, what initiated SIR2 normally presently couldn't seem to be found.

This is the place acetyl bunches become possibly the most important factor. It was at first idea that SIR2 may be a deacetylating compound — which means it expelled those acetyl gatherings — from different pbooks, yet nobody knew if this were valid since all endeavors to exhibit this movement in a test tube demonstrated negative. Guarente and his group had the option to find that SIR2 in yeast could just deacetylate different proteins within the sight of the coenzyme NAD+, nicotinamide adenine dinucleotide.

In Guarente's own words: "Without NAD+, SIR2 sits idle. That was the basic finding on the curve of sirtuin science."

Sirtuins inquire about has to a great extent been attached to maturing and metabolic action. "There are possibly 12,000 papers on sirtuins now," Guarente's said. "At the time we found the NAD+ subordinate deacetylase movement the quantity of papers was during the 100s."

As the sirtuins field keeps on growing, this leaves space for amazing exploration openings into how enacting sirtuins with NAD+ antecedents can prompt all the more energizing disclosures.

How to Fight the Excess Fat

Shock: Everyone has some gut fat, even individuals who have level abs.

That is typical. Be that as it may, a lot of tummy fat can influence your health such that other fat doesn't.

A portion of your fat is directly under your skin. Other fat is more profound inside, around your heart, lungs, liver, and different organs.

It's that more profound fat - called "instinctive" fat - that might be the more serious issue, in any event, for dainty individuals.

Profound Belly Fat

You need some instinctive fat. It gives padding around your organs.

However, if you have a lot of it, you might be bound to get hypertension, type 2 diabetes, coronary illness, dementia, and certain malignant growths, including bosom disease and colon disease.

The fat doesn't simply stay there. It's a functioning piece of your body, making "bunches of frightful substances," says Kristen Hairston, MD, right hand teacher of endocrinology and digestion at Wake Forest School of Medicine.

If you put on a lot of weight, your body begins to store your fat in bizarre spots.

With expanding heftiness, you have individuals whose ordinary zones to store fat are full to the point that the fat is kept into the organs and around the heart, says Carol Shively, PhD, teacher of pathology-similar medication at Wake Forest School of Medicine.

The amount Belly Fat Do You Have?

The most exact approach to decide how much instinctive fat you have is to get a CT sweep or MRI. Be that as it may, there's an a lot less difficult, ease approach to check.

Get an estimating tape, fold it over your abdomen at your midsection catch, and check your circumference. Do it while you're standing up, and ensure the measuring tape is level.

For the good of your health, you need your abdomen size to be under 35 inches if you're a lady and under 40 inches if you're a man.

Having a "pear shape" - greater hips and thighs - is viewed as more secure than an "apple shape," which portrays a more extensive waistline.

"What we're truly highlighting with the apple versus pear," Hairston says, "is that, if you have increasingly stomach fat, it's likely a marker that you have progressively instinctive fat."

Meager People Have It, Too

Regardless of whether you're slender, you can in any case have a lot of instinctive fat.

The amount you have is somewhat about your qualities, and halfway about your lifestyle, particularly how dynamic you are.

Instinctive fat preferences idleness. In one investigation, slight individuals who watched their diets yet didn't practice were bound to have an excessive amount of instinctive fat.

The key is to be dynamic, regardless of what size you are.

4 Steps for Beating Belly Fat

There are four keys to controlling paunch fat: work out, diet, rest, and stress the executives.

1. Exercise: Vigorous exercise cuts back the entirety of your excess, including instinctive fat.

Get at any rate 30 minutes of moderate exercise at any rate 5 days per week. Strolling tallies, as long as it's energetic enough that you burn some serious calories and inhale harder, with your pulse quicker than expected.

To get similar outcomes in a fraction of the time, step up your pace and get fiery exercise - like running or strolling. You'd have to do that for 20 minutes per day, 4 days every week.

Run, if you're now fit, or walk energetically at a slope on a treadmill if you're not prepared for running. Vivacious exercises on fixed bicycles and curved or paddling machines are additionally viable, says Duke analyst Cris Slentz, PhD.

Moderate movement - raising your pulse for 30 minutes at any rate three times each week - likewise makes a difference. It eases back down how much instinctive fat you gain. Be that as it may, to burn instinctive fat, your exercises ought to be ventured up.

"Rake leaves, walk, garden, go to Zumba, play soccer with your children. It doesn't need to be in the rec center," Hairston says.

If you are not dynamic currently, it's a smart thought to check with your health care supplier before beginning another workout schedule.

2. Diet: There is no enchantment diet for stomach fat. In any case, when you get fit on any diet, midsection fat as a rule goes first.

Getting enough fiber can help. Hairston's exploration shows that individuals who eat 10 grams of solvent fiber every day - with no other diet changes - develop less instinctive fat after some time than others. That is as basic as eating two little apples, a cup of green peas, or a half-cup of pinto beans.

"Regardless of whether you continued everything else the equivalent yet changed to a higher-fiber bread, you may have the option to all the more likely keep up your weight after some time," Hairston says.

3. Rest: Getting the perfect measure of shut-eye makes a difference. In one investigation, individuals who got 6 to 7 hours of rest for each night increased less instinctive fat more than 5 years contrasted with the individuals who dozed 5 or less hours out of every night or at least 8 hours out of every night. Rest might not have been the main thing that made a difference - however it was a piece of the image.

4. Stress: Everyone has pressure. How you handle it makes a difference. The best things you can do incorporate unwinding with loved ones, reflecting, practicing to let out some pent up frustration, and getting advising. That leaves you healthier and more ready to use sound judgment for yourself.

"If you could just bear the cost of an opportunity to do one of these things," Shively says, "practice presumably has the most prompt advantages, because it gets at both corpulence and stress."

CHAPTER 2: CASES STUDY

Aficionados of Grammy-winning songstress Adele, who simply commended her 32nd birthday, have been staying aware of Adele's weight loss through her Instagram profile since mid 2019. While the British chronicle craftsman has inconsistently posted pictures in the course of the most recent year, a spic and span post ending her months-long quietness on Instagram is becoming a web sensation for two reasons. First off, Adele is utilizing the chance to thank specialists on call: "I'd prefer to thank the entirety of our people on call and basic laborers who are protecting us while taking a chance with their lives! You are genuinely our holy messengers," she wrote in the image subtitle.

In any case, the post is additionally earning consideration likewise because of responses to her weight loss, including a message from Chrissy Teigen, who is a previous Sports Illustrated model herself: "I mean, are you messing with me," Chrissy remarked. Rita Wilson likewise really wanted to respond to the songstress' photograph: "Upbeat Birthday, Adele. Sending you so much love! Looking ravishing!"

It's just the most recent photograph to on the whole stagger the Internet, as Adele's continuous weight loss venture has provoked curiosity from inquisitive spectators throughout the most recent year. However, what fans can be sure of is that it appears Adele might be following an under-the-radar diet plan known as the Sirtfood Diet, which is intended to supercharge your digestion.

As indicated by People, Adele employed a fitness coach in 2019 to assist her with getting into another wellness schedule, however reports have since quite a while ago connected her weight loss to following the moderately new diet. She's lost in excess of 40 pounds by following the program in the course of the most recent four years, per The Sun (despite the fact that the artist hasn't affirmed any of this). What's more, she's by all account not the only Brit who depends on this diet, either — Pippa Middleton, the Duchess of Cambridge's sister, likewise allegedly has tried different things with the Sirtfood Diet.

While it absolutely may assist you with getting more fit, dieters might be shocked to discover that specialists aren't certain of the Sirtfood Diet's adequacy over the long haul. Here's the reason nutritionists are careful about the Sirtfood Diet in any case, and how you might have the option to adjust the best components of this prevailing fashion diet into your own.

In all honesty, this to some degree disputable diet program was propelled by two U.K.- based nutritionists, Aidan Goggins and Glen Matten, after they initially distributed a formula book by a similar name in 2016. The book touts the diet's adequacy as it turns on the "thin quality" by depending on staples that are high in sirtuins, a subset of plant-based proteins that can be found in specific foods and in the body normally. Expanded sirtuin levels in the body may help kick off your digestion and decrease aggravation, and has been featured for its enemy of maturing properties, as indicated by this 2013 survey distributed in the Annual Review of Physiology. "As a rule, it could be something worth being thankful for to eat foods that are rich in sirtuin — a quality that might have the option to help with weight — like apples, blueberries, and additional virgin olive oil," says Tracy Lockwood Beckerman, RD, creator of The Better Period Food Solution. Foods high in sirtuins, then, have been named "sirtfoods" in the diet plan.

As featured in The Official Sirtfood Diet, the diet program depends on a supper plan that is curated to be brimming with sirtfoods, however shortened in generally carbohydrate contents. Truth be told, one of the book's writers asserts that it can assist you with shedding seven pounds in a solitary week, as per the New York Post. In any case, the book's dinner plan is very controlled: For the initial three days, dieters are relied upon to devour only 1,000 calories every day that comprise of a solitary feast and two green juices. Later in the main week, dieters will appreciate 1,500-calorie dinner plans for four days that are for the most part partitioned between two suppers.

Most of the program requests that dieters make suppers that are high in sirtfoods... what more, very little else is. A portion of the staples that the diet feature incorporate various produce things, including kale, strawberries, onions, parsley, arugula, blueberries, and tricks. A few grains, similar to buckwheat, and pecans are applauded, as are flavors like turmeric. Strangely, refreshments like espresso, matcha green tea, and red wine are energized — similar to an overwhelming dependence on 85% dim chocolate.

If the diet's rundown of praised fixings appears to be somewhat deficient with regards to, you're not the only one — numerous health specialists reprimand the Sirtfood Diet for being exceptionally prohibitive.

41

Beckerman says she has never prescribed the Sirtfood Diet to any of her customers because of its tight calorie limitations. "While I acclaim the Sirtfood Diet for advancing the utilization of genuine fixings, I impugn it for its advancement of calorie limitation and unhealthy eating rules." Like numerous different diets that expel food bunches from normal utilization, Beckerman says the Sirtfood Diet may for sure lead to "confused eating" as it additionally mixes components from discontinuous fasting plans in with the general mish-mash.

McKenzie Caldwell, MPH, RDN, who spends significant time in ladies' sustenance and pregnancy dietary wellbeing specifically, says that the carbohydrate contents related with the diet are by a long shot it's most exceedingly awful quality. "1,000 calories for each day is just proper for a youngster between the ages of 2 and 4," she says, referring to current dietary rules circulated by the Mayo Clinic. "Not exclusively is this insufficient vitality to help a grown-up body, it is absurd to expect to fit in all the full scale and micronutrients a grown-up needs in that measure of food... The diet may cause weight loss in the present moment simply because of its caloric limitation."

Above all, notwithstanding, both sustenance specialists concur that there is practically zero clinical proof to help this diet being healthy for continued weight loss. "There is definitely no proof to back up any cases that the Sirtfood Diet beneficially affects healthy weight loss," Beckerman says. "The makers of the diet guarantee to have put members at their own exercise center on the diet, however this recounted assumed examination has not been distributed nor approved by evident specialists or researchers."

Much the same as Keto and Whole30, the Sirtfood Diet often radicalizes how you ordinarily eat by requesting that you hold back on dinners. While all diets often stick to some type of a calorie-limit, Caldwell says it's essential to consider your own lifestyle and consider what you need for the duration of the day. "Actually, there is nothing mysterious about sirtfoods specifically — being rich in polyphenols, they do have calming properties, however the exploration doesn't bolster them having any additional viability for weight loss."

If you're hell bent on checking out the Sirtfood Diet, first examination by consolidating a greater amount of the diet's mark staples into what you're now eating at home. "Consolidating polyphenol-rich foods, including those on the sirtfood list, can be useful in forestalling or lessening fiery ailments like cardiovascular infection," she prompts. "Avoid the underlying prohibitive advances and endorsed green juices, and rather select including cell reinforcement rich foods to your eating design in a manner you appreciate."

CHAPTER 3: THE FIRST PHASE: 7 POUNDS IN 7 DAYS

Regardless of whether you have an uncommon event coming up or are flying off to a sea shore occasion one week from now, we have the ideal healthy eating intend to assist you with shedding pounds rapidly.

So would you be able to get thinner in seven days? With the multi week diet plan, you could lose as much as seven pounds in seven days.

Getting trim can be precarious and attempting to get in shape quick can be considerably increasingly difficult. Time after time, we promise to head out to the rec center each morning and stay alive on only one low-cal dinner every day, just to wind up coming up short and gorging on cake and chocolate on day two. That is because prevailing fashion diets can be unimaginably prohibitive and often leave us feeling ravenous and unsatisfied – also ailing in vitality.

No more! With the multi week diet plan, you can get in shape quick and feel extraordinary in only seven days – without starving yourself en route. Win big or bust diets set you up for disappointment, however the multi week diet plan permits you to eat three full dinners for every days, including loads of healthy foods grown from the ground, in addition to eating in the middle of suppers.

You'll feel full and fulfilled, on account of the high protein admission and a lot of fiber-filled vegetables and organic products. Sugar is off the menu yet don't stress, you're despite everything permitted your day by day espresso or tea fix – simply ensure it's decaf!

There are no contrivances to the multi week diet, simply brilliant guidance and simple to-adhere to guidelines. The weight loss plan is low in fat, low in carbs, however high in bravo foods. What's more, best of all, dinners can be put together quick, making the diet significantly simpler to adhere to!

If you're intending to shift the pounds in only seven days, it's critical to tolerate as a primary concern that it won't be simple, and that you'll need to keep up a confined diet so as to see the advantages.

So as to get in shape in such a little space of time, you'll have to keep your carbohydrate content low, while as yet keeping up a healthy diet plan that will keep you fulfilled – as, obviously, you're bound to need the awful stuff if you aren't!

Step by step instructions to get thinner in seven days: The dinner plans

Regardless of whether you have an uncommon event coming up or are flying off to a sea shore occasion one week from now, we have the ideal healthy eating intend to assist you with shedding pounds quick. Indeed, with the multi week diet plan, you could lose as much as seven pounds in seven days!

Shedding pounds can be difficult and attempting to shed pounds quick can feel practically unimaginable. Over and over again, we promise to go to the exercise center each morning and attempt to remain alive on only one low-cal feast every day, just to wind up coming up short and gorging on cake and chocolate on day two.

That is because trend diets can be fantastically prohibitive and often leave us feeling ravenous and unsatisfied – also ailing in vitality. No more! With the multi week diet plan, you can get in shape and feel incredible in only seven days – without starving yourself en route.

There are no contrivances to the multi week diet, simply savvy exhortation and simple to-adhere to directions. The weight loss plan is low in fat, low in carbs however high in bravo foods. Best of all, suppers can be put together quick, making the diet significantly simpler to adhere to!

Win or bust diets set you up for disappointment. In any case, the multi week diet plan permits you to eat three full suppers for each days, including bunches of healthy foods grown from the ground, in addition to eating in the middle of dinners. You'll feel full and fulfilled, on account of the high protein admission and a lot of nutritious foods. Sugar is off the menu however don't stress, you're despite everything permitted your day by day espresso or tea fix – simply ensure it's decaf!

Breakfast

Oats, organic product, low fat yogurt would all be able to fill in as a healthy breakfast in all structures. You could assemble them all in a bowl, or whisk them up to make a yummy smoothie.

Eggs and greens are likewise an incredible method to begin your day if you're intending to lose a decent lot of weight in a short space of time. Attempt an omelette, fried egg and avocado on toast, or a straightforward poached or bubbled egg with veggies like asparagus as an afterthought.

Recollect that morning meal is the most significant feast of the day, so don't ration the parts!

Your day by day diet: Morning nibble

Organic product - new and as much as you can imagine. Make a major organic product serving of mixed greens, mix into a smoothie or eat the entire natural product if you have to eat on the run. A banana is additionally a smart thought - so as to top you off until noon.

Notwithstanding, don't have excessively near lunch however - leave at any rate an hour hole to help assimilation.

Lunch

A major plate of mixed greens of anything you extravagant is a good thought. Include a little part of protein - possibly fish or chicken about the size of a deck of cards. Furthermore, treat yourself to a sprinkle of olive oil and lemon.

Steer away from terrible fats, for example, cheddar and pasta, yet be liberable with the great fats - avocado and yam are extraordinary.

Whole wheat wraps, or pitta brimming with plate of mixed greens and protein are likewise an incredible alternative for your late morning supper. Obviously, for the colder days, hand crafted soups are a decent decision as well - as they're low in calories.

Your day by day diet: Afternoon nibble

No curve balls here, however the most ideal approach if you'd prefer to get thinner in only seven days is with more leafy foods a little bunch of seeds - sunflower or pumpkin are your most logical option and they're anything but difficult to purchase. Or then again if you can eat with restriction, attempt a couple of pecans or almonds. They're higher in fat, yet with some restraint, are extraordinary for you.

Supper

A super enormous plate of mixed greens with bunches of intriguing 'substantial' things like beetroot or avocado – not simply leaves! - is a decent choice. Include a bigger part of protein this time (attempt a chicken bosom or a container of salmon). Also dressing as in the past.

You can likewise permit yourself some moderate discharge carbs by this point in the day - attempt and straightforward chicken and rice dish, or a salmon and yam dinner. Little parts of entire wheat pasta or a lean steak with the fat cut off can likewise function admirably.

Fish is additionally a strong decision when it comes to settling on supper choices, however ensure that you're continually picking the new choice - cod, haddock, and so forth - instead of its battered variant.

The beverages

Parts and heaps of water is prompted, ideally two or three liters per day at any rate. In addition, you can permit yourself some home grown teas and dark decaff espresso or tea. It's simply too coldblooded to even think about depriving yourself of these separation the-day hot beverages!

So what CAN'T you eat?

You presumably needn't bother with us to reveal to you this, however during your week diet, it's ideal to avoid refined starches, for example, baked goods, white bread, white pasta, or potatoes.

Similarly, it's indispensable that you avoid sugar in the entirety of its structures - regardless of whether in a bundle of desserts or in a sweet bubbly beverage.

What's more, on the subject of beverages, when you're attempting to get in shape, it's consistently a smart thought to skip liquor! Indeed - even that gin and tonic you were told had no calories.

51

We know, it's extreme. Be that as it may, when you think about your new certain bodies, will undoubtedly merit all the difficult work.

Without paying, as far as anyone is concerned there are not many if any projects like this that give you the specifics to get in shape in seven days.

Fortunately I'm going to impart all that to you for literally nothing. Because I can. So I trust you appreciate it and give it your everything.

Here's the manner by which it will work. I'll go through some fundamental tips and deceives that you'll have to begin doing to quicken your weight loss before giving you the diet plan and exercises with recordings.

It will be essential yet then this is the free form for the 6 Week Flat Belly Challenge however I guarantee you it will be very powerful and exactly what you have to lose as much as 7 pounds in the following 7 days.

1. Quit EATING PROCESSED FOODS

From now and the following 7 days you won't permit anything prepared or artificial pass your lips. These foods will in general be exceptionally high in poisons and soaked fats which will make you store undesirable fat.

You ought to have the option to know whether a food is handled yet when in question check the fixings mark. If the item being referred to has multiple fixings it's conceivable prepared.

The special cases would be if it was a pre marinade chicken bosom or almond milk for instance.

The main foods you can devour must be in their entire common structure. The closer to that the better.

It's only 7 days, you are free to plan for a cheat feast toward the finish of your 7 days, after your say something obviously.

Your dinners should comprise of a protein source, for example, eggs, salmon or chicken, a few vegetables and maybe some dietary fat from avocado.

2. NO MORE ALCOHOL

It's an ideal opportunity to lose some weight, I challenge you to shed 7 pounds in the following 7 days and I'll even give all of you the instruments you have to take care of business. The 7 Day Challenge. Lose 7 lbs in seven days

Liquor will prevent you from shedding pounds. When you devour liquor your body will incidentally quit processing different supplements, for example, fat. It additionally impedes the assimilation of supplements, for example, proteins, significant for muscle fix after your HIIT exercises.

For the following 7 days, no more liquor. Spare it for day 8 if you should.

3. GET 7-8 HOURS SLEEP

Being drained is connected to expanded yearning, something you will need to attempt to abstain from during any weight loss challenge except if you are amazingly solid willed.

Absence of rest additionally adjusts your degrees of Cortisol, a hormone that will make you store midsection fat. Raised levels won't assist you with disposing of midsection fat, which is guaranteed. So attempt your best to head to sleep a better than average time. I feel like your folks, sorry. 7-8 hours is generally a decent beginning, just you realize the amount you truly need.

Our primary strategic to ensure you get enough rest so you wake up feeling stimulated and prepared to have an incredible day.

4. YOU'RE GOING TO CUT THOSE CARBS

It's a great opportunity to lose some weight, I challenge you to shed 7 pounds in the following 7 days and I'll even give all of you the instruments you have to take care of business. The 7 Day Challenge. Lose 7 lbs in seven days

Indeed, the carbs need to descend. For quick fat loss, we have to get your body consuming fat and lose some water weight from the put away glycogen.

Evacuating or diminishing your starch admission including sugar you will give your body an incredible opportunity to begin consuming fat as its essential fuel source. Our diet does even now permit starches with one supper daily, in a perfect world on preparing days. This will be clarified more inside the 7 Day Challenge itself.

5. EXERCISE

It's an ideal opportunity to lose some weight, I challenge you to shed 7 pounds in the following 7 days and I'll even give all of you the instruments you have to take care of business. The 7 Day Challenge. Lose 7 lbs in seven days

You can diminish your calorie admission by eating less and increment your action levels to consume more calories. In the multi day Challenge, we do both to amplify your weight loss potential.

Just as the High Intensity Interval Training exercises gave in the 7 Day Challenge I need you to stroll for 45 minutes per day.

The point of the strolling is to let your body let loose fat cells and use it for vitality. In a perfect world, you will stroll in the mornings for the sole quick that once it's done it's done and you won't need to stress over accomplishing it after work or school, you can simply focus on your food.

6. WATER

Ultimately on our top tips for quick weight loss is to ensure you are getting a lot of liquids from water.

Being all around hydrated will permit your body to work better and along these lines digestion vitality all the more effectively.

You'll be progressively engaged and have more vitality which will prompt better exercises and less compulsion to eat severely.

Focus on 2-3 liters of water spread for the duration of the day.

THE 7 DAY CHALLENGE

So here it is, The 7 Day Challenge that will direct you through quick weight loss.

We've structured a simple to follow multi day eating plan with plans and a read it and eat it intend to kick you off.

Likewise included is the most, exercises. In the arrangement, you have two exercises with recordings to help quicken your fat loss.

To get to the diet plan and exercises click the catch beneath or here.

It will take you to a login page where you have to make a sign in to get your hands on the plans.

"I need more time," is the most established weight-loss pardon in the book, and it's actually what my companion, Jenny, let me know as we strolled through the rancher's market last Sunday.

"All things considered, do you have sufficient opportunity to eat?" I asked her.

"Better believe it," she said.

"Then you're out of reasons!" I replied. With the correct direction—and the correct outlook—you can soften fat and accelerate digestion by essentially tweaking certain propensities. Make these seven changes to your day by day schedule on Sunday, and you'll be seven pounds more slender by Saturday! (That is extraordinary news for you: In one investigation, the individuals who shed 15 percent of their body weight inside the initial a half year of their diets are the most drastically averse to recapture the weight.) So begin getting thinner today—

and make a point to consistently maintain a strategic distance from these 50 Little Things Making You Fatter and Fatter.

Ever understand that attempting to make sense of what you're going to make for supper that equivalent night often brings about getting a pizza or eating Goober Grape directly from the container? Plan heretofore, and do a brisk shop. Since home cooks devour a normal of 140 calories less per dinner, you'll be an entire pound lighter if you try preparing every supper at home this week.

Eat This! Tip:

The best dieters use a supper topic recipe and basically pivot only a couple go-to dinners and bites. Figure: Meatless Monday can be both southwestern quinoa skillet and pasta primavera while Crockpot Saturday includes a tasty pork carnitas and liquefy in-your mouth pot broil (or any of these 35 Delicious One-Pot Slow Cooker Recipes).

Breakfast is the most significant supper of the day for an explanation: An investigation distributed in Obesity Research and Clinical Practice demonstrated that eating a morning feast assists dieters with keeping up progressively predictable blood glucose levels; subsequently, you'll have increasingly stable vitality levels for the duration of the day and won't need to whip those growling food cravings into their place. While we know not every person has an entire hour to prepare a morning meal buffet, that doesn't mean you need to pass up a spread of craving busting, fat-battling supplements. Simply get a smoothie!

Eat This! Tip:

Our go to is the Ginger Man Smoothie from our top of the line book, Zero Belly Smoothies. The solidified strawberries are abounding with nutrient C to help assault paunch fat-putting away Cortisol levels, newly ground ginger's gingerol combined with banana's potassium will help debloat your tummy, the omega-3s in ground flaxseed will battle off weight-instigating irritation, and the plant-based protein powder will give 29 grams of backbone to keep you full until lunch.

Consider it: for what reason do you truly decide to get that pack of Cheetos from the candy machine? Is it because you realize they'll fulfill your yearning longings?

(They won't.) Or is it because you don't have something else? We'd put down our wagers on the subsequent one. Tidbits are an extraordinary method to feed your digestion and feed your mind, yet they'll possibly help if they're of the "healthy" assortment. What's more, prepare to be blown away. Accommodation is an immense factor here. Indeed, it might be the main factor. When Northwestern University specialists supplanted low quality nourishment with healthy choices in Chicago park candy machines, not exclusively did 88 percent of those studied report getting a charge out of the tidbits, however deals additionally expanded by a stunning 340 percent! So try finding out about these Meal Prep Sunday Tips, and prepare your food to get in a hurry.

Eat This! Tip:

From buying new organic product to leave on your counter, to slicing up veggies to keep in your refrigerator, to stirring up some moment cereal combos, the opportunities for inexpensive food are perpetual!

CHAPTER 4: THE SECOND PHASE: MAINTENANCE

Sadly, numerous individuals who shed pounds wind up recovering it.

Truth be told, just about 20% of dieters who start off overweight end up effectively getting more fit and keeping it off in the long haul.

Be that as it may, don't let this debilitate you. There are various scientifically demonstrated ways you can keep the weight off, running from practicing to controlling pressure.

These 17 techniques may be exactly what you have to tip the insights in support of you and keep up your hard-won weight loss.

Why People Regain Weight

There are a couple of basic reasons why individuals restore the weight they lose. They are generally identified with ridiculous desires and sentiments of hardship.

Prohibitive diets: Extreme calorie limitation may slow your digestion and shift your craving managing hormones, which are the two factors that add to weight recover.

Wrong mentality: When you think about a diet as a convenient solution, instead of a drawn out answer for better your health, you will be bound to surrender and restore the weight you lost.

Absence of supportable propensities: Many diets depend on self control instead of propensities you can consolidate into your day by day life. They center on rules as opposed to lifestyle changes, which may dishearten you and forestall weight support.

Synopsis:

Numerous diets are excessively prohibitive with necessities that are difficult to stay aware of. Furthermore, numerous individuals don't have the correct outlook before beginning a diet, which may prompt weight recapture.

1. Exercise Often

Customary exercise assumes a significant job in weight support.

It might assist you with consuming off some additional calories and increment your digestion, which are two variables expected to accomplish vitality balance.

When you are in vitality balance, it implies you consume a similar number of calories that you devour. Subsequently, your weight is bound to remain the equivalent.

A few examinations have discovered that individuals who do at any rate 200 minutes of moderate physical movement seven days (30 minutes every day) in the wake of getting thinner are bound to keep up their weight.

In certain occurrences, much more significant levels of physical movement might be essential for fruitful weight support. One survey reasoned that one hour of activity daily is ideal for those endeavoring to keep up weight loss.

Note that activity is the most supportive for weight upkeep when it's joined with other lifestyle changes, including adhering to a healthy diet.

Rundown:

Practicing for at any rate 30 minutes of the day may advance weight support by helping balance your calories in and calories consumed.

2. Take a stab at Eating Breakfast Every Day

Having breakfast may help you with your weight upkeep objectives.

Breakfast eaters will in general have healthier propensities by and large, for example, practicing more and expending more fiber and micronutrients.

Besides, having breakfast is one of the most widely recognized practices announced by people who are effective at keeping up weight loss.

One examination found that 78% of 2,959 individuals who kept up a 30-pound (14 kg) weight loss for at any rate one year announced having breakfast each day.

Be that as it may, while individuals who have breakfast appear to be fruitful at keeping up weight loss, the proof is blended.

Studies don't show that skipping breakfast consequently prompts weight addition or more terrible dietary patterns.

Indeed, skipping breakfast may even assist some with peopling accomplish their weight loss and weight upkeep objectives.

This might be something that comes down to the person.

If you feel that having breakfast encourages you adhere to your objectives, then you unquestionably ought to eat it. Be that as it may, if you don't care for having breakfast or are not eager toward the beginning of the day, there is no mischief in skipping it.

Rundown:

The individuals who have breakfast will have healthier propensities by and large, which may assist them with keeping up their weight. In any case, skipping breakfast doesn't naturally prompt weight gain.

3. Eat Lots of Protein

Eating a great deal of protein may assist you with keeping up your weight, since protein can help decrease craving and advance totality.

Protein expands levels of specific hormones in the body that incite satiety and are significant for weight guideline. Protein has additionally been appeared to lessen levels of hormones that expansion hunger.

Protein's impact on your hormones and totality may naturally decrease the quantity of calories you devour every day, which is a significant factor in weight support.

Besides, protein requires a significant measure of vitality for your body to separate. Therefore, eating it normally may build the quantity of calories you consume during the day.

In view of a few investigations, apparently protein's impacts on digestion and hunger are most unmistakable when about 30% of calories are devoured from protein. This is 150 grams of protein on a 2,000 calorie diet.

Rundown:

Protein may profit weight support by advancing completion, expanding digestion and decreasing your absolute calorie admission.

4. Gauge Yourself Regularly

Observing your weight by stepping on the scale all the time might be a useful device for weight upkeep. This is because it can gain you mindful of your ground and energize weight control practices.

The individuals who gauge themselves may likewise eat less calories for the duration of the day, which is useful for keeping up weight loss.

Overall, expended 300 less calories for each day than the individuals who observed their weight less regularly.

How often you gauge yourself is an individual decision. Some think that it's supportive to say something every day, while others are progressively effective checking their weight on more than one occasion per week.

Outline:

Self-weighing may help weight upkeep by keeping you mindful of your advancement and practices.

5. Be Mindful of Your Carb Intake

Weight upkeep might be simpler to achieve if you focus on the sorts and measures of carbs that you eat.

Eating too many refined carbs, for example, white bread, white pasta and natural product juices, can be inconvenient to your weight upkeep objectives.

These foods have been deprived of their regular fiber, which is important to advance totality. Diets that are low in fiber are related with weight addition and heftiness.

Constraining your carb admission generally speaking may likewise assist you with keeping up your weight loss. A few investigations have discovered that, now and again, the individuals who follow low-carb diets after weight loss are bound to keep the weight off in the long haul.

Moreover, individuals following low-carb diets are more averse to eat a larger number of calories than they consume, which is essential for weight upkeep.

Outline:

Restricting your admission of carbs, particularly those that are refined, may help forestall weight recover.

6. Lift Weights

Diminished bulk is a typical reaction of weight loss.

It can constrain your capacity to keep weight off, as losing muscle decreases your digestion, which means you consume less calories for the duration of the day (34).

Doing some kind of obstruction preparing, for example, lifting weights, may help forestall this loss of muscle and, thus, safeguard or even improve your metabolic rate.

Studies show that the individuals who lift weights after weight loss are bound to keep weight off by keeping up bulk.

To get these advantages, it is prescribed to take part in quality preparing in any event two times every week. Your preparation routine should work all muscle bunches for ideal outcomes.

Outline:

Lifting weights in any event two times every week may help with weight upkeep by saving your bulk, which is essential to support a healthy digestion.

7. Be Prepared for Setbacks

Misfortunes are inescapable on your weight support venture. There might be times when you surrender to an unhealthy needing or skirt an exercise.

In any case, the periodic foul up doesn't mean you should toss your objectives out the window. Essentially proceed onward and finish better decisions.

It can likewise assist with preparing for circumstances that you realize will make healthy eating testing, for example, an up and coming get-away or occasion.

Outline:

Almost certainly, you will experience a misfortune or two in the wake of getting in shape. You can beat misfortunes by preparing and refocusing immediately.

8. Adhere to Your Plan All Week Long (Even on Weekends)

One propensity that often prompts weight recapture is eating healthy on weekdays and undermining ends of the week.

This attitude often drives individuals to gorge on low quality nourishment, which can balance weight support endeavors.

If it turns into a normal propensity, you could recover more weight than you lost in any case.

Then again, inquire about shows that the individuals who follow a reliable eating design all during the time are bound to continue weight loss in the long haul.

One investigation found that week after week consistency made people twice as prone to keep up their weight inside five pounds (2.2 kg) more than one year, contrasted with the individuals who permitted greater adaptability on the ends of the week.

Synopsis:

Fruitful weight upkeep is simpler to achieve when you adhere to your healthy dietary patterns throughout the entire week, remembering for ends of the week.

9. Remain Hydrated

Drinking water is useful for weight upkeep for a couple of reasons.

First of all, it advances completion and may assist you with holding your calorie consumption within proper limits if you drink a glass or two preceding suppers.

In one investigation, the individuals who drank water before eating a supper had a 13% decrease in calorie consumption, contrasted with members who didn't drink water.

Furthermore, drinking water has been appeared to somewhat build the quantity of calories you consume for the duration of the day.

Rundown:

Drinking water normally may advance completion and increment your digestion, both significant factors in weight upkeep.

10. Get Enough Sleep

Getting enough rest significantly influences weight control.

Actually, lack of sleep gives off an impression of being a significant hazard factor for weight gain in grown-ups and may meddle with weight upkeep.

This is incompletely because of the way that deficient rest prompts more elevated levels of ghrelin, which is known as the craving hormone because it builds hunger.

In addition, poor sleepers will in general have lower levels of leptin, which is a hormone vital for hunger control.

Besides, the individuals who rest for brief timeframes are essentially worn out and therefore less spurred to exercise and settle on healthy food decisions.

If you're not resting enough, figure out how to change your rest propensities. Resting for at any rate seven hours a night is ideal for weight control and generally health.

Resting for healthy time spans may help with weight support by keeping your vitality step up and hormones leveled out.

11. Control Stress Levels

Overseeing pressure is a significant piece of controlling your weight.

Truth be told, high feelings of anxiety can add to weight recapture by expanding levels of Cortisol, which is a hormone discharged in light of pressure.

Reliably raised Cortisol is connected to higher measures of stomach fat, just as expanded craving and food admission.

Stress is additionally a typical trigger for indiscreet eating, which is when you eat in any event, when you're not eager.

Luckily, there are numerous things you can never really stretch, including activity, yoga and reflection.

Rundown:

It is imperative to monitor feelings of anxiety to keep up your weight, as overabundance stress may build the danger of weight gain by animating your craving.

12. Discover a Support System

It tends to be difficult to keep up your weight objectives alone.

One procedure to defeat this is to discover an emotionally supportive network that will consider you responsible and perhaps accomplice up with you in your healthy lifestyle.

A couple of studies have demonstrated that having a mate to seek after your objectives with might be useful for weight control, particularly if that individual is an accomplice or life partner with comparable healthy propensities.

One of these examinations analyzed the health practices of more than 3,000 couples and found that when one individual occupied with a healthy propensity, for example, work out, the other was bound to follow their model.

Outline:

Including an accomplice or companion in your healthy lifestyle may support the probability that you will keep up your weight loss.

13. Track Your Food Intake

The individuals who log their food admission in a diary, online food tracker or application might be bound to keep up their weight loss.

Food trackers are useful because they upgrade your attention to the amount you are truly eating, since they often give specific data about what number of calories and supplements you expend.

Moreover, numerous food-following instruments permit you to log work out, so you can guarantee you're getting the sum you have to keep up your weight.

Here are a few instances of calorie checking sites and applications.

Outline:

Logging your food consumption from everyday may assist you with keeping up your weight loss by making you mindful of what number of calories and supplements you're eating.

14. Eat Plenty of Vegetables

A few investigations connect high vegetable admission to all the more likely weight control.

First of all, vegetables are low in calories. You can eat enormous segments without gaining weight, while as yet expending a noteworthy measure of supplements.

Additionally, vegetables are high in fiber, which builds sentiments of completion and may naturally diminish the quantity of calories that you eat during the day.

For these weight control benefits, mean to devour a serving or two of vegetables at each feast.

Vegetables are high in fiber and low in calories. Both of these properties might be useful for weight support.

15. Be Consistent

Consistency is critical to keeping weight off.

Rather than on-and-off dieting that closes with returning to old propensities, it is ideal to stay with your new healthy diet and lifestyle for good.

While receiving another lifestyle may appear to be overpowering from the start, settling on healthy decisions will turn out to be natural when you become accustomed to them.

Your healthier lifestyle will be easy, so you'll have the option to keep up your weight substantially more without any problem.

Keeping up weight loss is straightforward when you are steady with your new healthy propensities, as opposed to returning to your old lifestyle.

16. Practice Mindful Eating

Careful eating is the act of tuning in to inward hunger signals and giving full consideration during the eating procedure.

It includes eating gradually, without interruptions, and biting food completely so you can relish the smell and taste of your dinner.

When you eat along these lines, you are bound to quit eating when you are genuinely full. If you eat while diverted, it very well may be difficult to perceive totality and you may wind up indulging.

Studies show that careful eating assists with weight support by focusing on practices that are ordinarily connected with weight increase, for example, passionate eating.

Additionally, the individuals who eat carefully might have the option to keep up their weight without checking calories.

Outline:

Careful eating is useful for weight upkeep because it encourages you perceive completion and may forestall unhealthy practices that generally lead to weight gain.

17. Roll out Sustainable Improvements to Your Lifestyle

The motivation behind why numerous individuals fall flat at keeping up their weight is because they follow unreasonable diets that are not doable in the long haul.

They wind up feeling denied, which often prompts restoring more weight than they lost in any case once they return to eating regularly.

Keeping up weight loss comes down to rolling out supportable improvements to your lifestyle.

This appears to be unique for everybody, except basically it implies not being excessively prohibitive, remaining predictable and settling on healthy decisions as often as could be expected under the circumstances.

It is simpler to keep up weight loss when you make reasonable lifestyle changes, instead of observing the ridiculous standards that many weight loss diets center around.

The Bottom Line

Diets can be prohibitive and unreasonable, which often prompts weight recover.

In any case, there are a lot of straightforward changes you can make to your propensities that are anything but difficult to stay with and will assist you with keeping up your weight loss in the long haul.

Through your excursion, you will understand that controlling your weight includes substantially more than what you eat. Exercise, rest and psychological wellness additionally assume a job.

It is workable for weight support to be easy if you basically embrace another lifestyle, instead of going on and off weight loss diets.

CHAPTER 5: TOP SIRTFOODS

Buckwheat

Escapades

Celery

Bean stew

Chocolate

Espresso

Additional Virgin Olive Oil

Green Tea – preferably matcha

Kale

Lovage

Medjool Dates

Parsley

Red Chicory

Red Onion

Red Wine

Rocket

Soy

Strawberries

Turmeric

Pecans

Only a token of the scientific foundation to the Sirtfood diet plan...

Sirtfoods are the notable methods for enacting our sirtuin qualities in the most ideal manner. These are the marvel foods especially wealthy in specific characteristic plant synthetic concoctions, called polyphenols, which have the ability to enact our sirtuin qualities by turning them on. Basically, they mirror the impacts of fasting and practice and in doing so bring exceptional advantages by helping the body to all the more likely control glucose levels, consume fat, form muscle and lift health and memory.

Because they're fixed, plants have built up a profoundly complex pressure reaction framework and produce polyphenols to assist them with adjusting to the difficulties of their condition. When we devour these plants, we likewise expend these polyphenol supplements. Their impact is significant: they actuate our own intrinsic pressure reaction pathways.

While all plants have pressure reaction frameworks, just certain ones have created to deliver imperative measures of sirtuin-initiating polyphenols. These plants are sirtfoods. Their revelation implies that rather than exacting fasting regimens or challenging activity programs, there's presently a progressive better approach to initiate your sirtuin qualities: eating a diet bottomless in sirtfoods. The best part is that the diet includes putting (sirt) foods onto your plate, not taking them off.

CHAPTER 6: DIET PLANS

In light of these standards, this is what could be on the menu longer than seven days during the support stage (green squeezes aside).

Breakfast

Kale omelet

Muesli, yogurt and blueberries

Organic product smoothie made with moved oats and soy milk

Lunch and supper

Rocket plate of mixed greens with fish, tomatoes and cucumber wearing olive oil

Veggie-stuffed hot tofu pan sear with winged creatures eye bean stew

Barbecued fish with buckwheat serving of mixed greens

Chicken and soba noodle pan sear

Tofu burgers with wholegrain bread and serving of mixed greens

Kale serving of mixed greens with edamame beans and red onion wearing olive oil

Fiery chicken curry presented with wholegrain earthy colored rice

Tidbits

Espresso

Celery and hummus

New organic product, especially strawberries, apples and oranges

Pecans

Dim chocolate

Sirtfood diet warnings to remember

With everything taken into account, the Sirtfood diet doesn't appear to be really awful from the unaided eye. Yet, as a dietitian, I have a couple of significant issue.

To begin, with I'm not a devotee of the extraordinary limitation toward the beginning of stage one. The possibility that this stage detoxifies your body is simply babble – your organs are more than equipped for doing only that.

Furthermore, living on just 1000 calories daily is *really* difficult work. Unremitting food cravings are too awkward, also the effect that could have on your public activity. You most likely won't have the option to meet your every day supplement prerequisites during this stage, either, because of the general absence of food. Obviously, there are advantages to irregular fasting, however it's not for everybody.

The very certainty this is a 'diet' is another explanation I wouldn't suggest it. The extreme food rules will turn out to be too difficult to even consider sticking to – so you'll likely surrender, feel remorseful and afterward start the diet again, and keep on rehashing this cycle however never truly go anyplace.

It likewise truly granulates my apparatuses when diets like this set a few foods up in place of worship as though they're an enchantment shot – truth is, all foods can and ought to be a piece of a healthy diet. What's significant is assortment, instead of expending a lot of a couple of select foods.

If weight loss is your objective, I'd urge you to channel your vitality into making practical lifestyle transforms you can adhere to, for good – instead of burning through your time with senseless eating plans like the Sirtfood diet.

You may have known about the Sirtfood Plan previously - particularly since it was accounted for vocalist Adele lost 50lbs after the arrangement - however do you know what it really is?

The eating plan characterizes the 20 foods that turn on your supposed 'thin qualities', boosting your digestion and your vitality levels. Truth be told, it specifies that you could lose 7lbs in 7 days...

The eating plan will change the manner in which you do healthy eating. It might seem like a non-easy to understand name, however it's one you'll be catching wind of a great deal.

Because the 'Sirt' in Sirtfoods is shorthand for the sirtuin qualities, a gathering of qualities nicknamed the 'thin qualities' that work, to be perfectly honest, similar to enchantment.

Eating these foods, state the makers of the arrangement, nutritionists Aidan Goggins and Glen Matten, turns on these qualities and "copies the impacts of calorie limitation, fasting and exercise". It initiates a reusing procedure in the body, "that gets out the cell trash and mess which amasses after some time and causes sick health and loss of imperativeness,"

These foods contain significant levels of plant synthetic concoctions called polyphenols, which are thought to turn on the Sirtuin qualities thus incite their super-healthy advantages.

The main 20 Sirtfoods incorporate red wine, cocoa (dim chocolate!) and espresso. Buckwheat is the fundamental carb on the rundown, and such was the achievement of the main book – The Sirtfood Diet – when it propelled a year ago, that health food shops sold out of it, and buckwheat noodle maker Clearspring needed to twofold its creation.

To test in the case of eating foods high in sirtuins has a beneficial outcome, the group checked the advancement of a little sample of 40 rec center goers.

Every one of the members lost 7lbs in seven days and detailed more significant levels of vitality.

A creature concentrate in 2012 indicated how a sirtuin called Sirt6 lengthened the lifespan of male mice by 15.8 percent, while later research demonstrated that Sirt1 is connected to a healthier digestion in mice took care of a high-fat diet.

In any case, an ongoing report by the Journal of Physiology additionally indicated that eating sirtuin-rich food could make practice less viable at bringing down circulatory strain and controlling cholesterol. Be that as it may, this examination included elevated levels of sirtuin supplements, at 250mg per day, the Telegraph detailed.

In this way, the impacts of the eating foods containing sirtuins will be better comprehended with further examination.

There are two periods of the sirtfood diet, with stage one enduring seven days. For this first week, days one through three are constrained to 1,000 calories for each day and incorporate three sirtfood-affirmed green juices and one dinner. After the third day, you can devour

1,500 calories for each day as two green juices and two dinners. In a report by USA Today, it clarifies that the second period of the sirtfood diet endures 14 days and incorporates "three suppers high in sirtfoods, one sirtfood green juice, and a couple sirtfood nibble snacks."

CHAPTER 7: QUESTIONS & ANSWERS

Sounds unrealistic, we know, however with red wine and dull chocolate on the menu, the Sirtfood Diet as of now has armies of adherents and is set to overwhelm the diet world.

What is the Sirtfood diet?

"They suggest eating specific foods which are very health foods, for example, kale, soy, additionally red wine for instance. In any case, they do likewise promoter to limit calories. So what they state is to eat around 1000 calories every day for the initial three days and afterward stick to around 1500 calories. So if you're taking that measure of calories, you are probably going to shed pounds."

For what reason is it engaging?

"If I reveal to you that you can have your dim chocolate and your wine, I believe are bound to follow that diet because you will be ready to eat things you appreciate."

Is it safe?

"Hard to learn if it's sheltered or not because there aren't any examinations that have taken a gander at the diet long haul. What's more, if you do limit yourself the sum they advocate like a 1000 calories every day, which is certainly undependable, particularly if you're not in a restoratively administered condition."

What is worried about the Sirtfood diet?

Dr. Viana says — drinking red wine. "While we believe it's reasonable safe for ladies to have one beverage daily and men to have two beverages per day, numerous individuals that have weight, may likewise have liver infection that they don't think about and that measure of liquor admission, despite the fact that perhaps healthy, if you have a basic liver malady, it may be a lot for you."

Any Celebrity fans?

James Haskell, Jodie Kidd and Lorraine Pascale, to give some examples.

The TV cook says: "A non-faddy diet that offers mind boggling health advantages and weight loss. Aidan and Glen show how everybody can receive the rewards of the Sirtfood Diet through eating scrumptious food. I'm a gigantic fan!"

What amount of will I lose?

Goggins and Matten's tests at an European health club demonstrated the normal dieter to lose 7lbs in 7 days, and an expansion in bulk and general prosperity. What's the trick? Research on the health advantages of 'sirtfoods' is still in its initial days, so while the diet is extraordinary for empowering utilization of products of the soil, you might be baffled if you're searching for emotional weight loss.

Likewise, the tests performed on exercise center individuals saw the members devour around 1,000 calories for the initial three days, then 1,500 for the rest of the days, proposing that it's essential to lessen generally speaking calorie utilization just as joining 'sirtfoods' into your diet.

With big names, for example, Adele and Pippa Middleton said to have bounced on the Sirtfood Diet train, it has everybody intrigued asking how does the Sirtfood Diet work precisely. Advanced for bringing "powerful and supported weight loss", the diet is tied in with eating certain foods that will "initiate" one's "thin quality". Food Network separates it that the entirety of the foods recorded above contain a "characteristic substance called polyphenols that mirrors the impacts of activity and fasting".

If one adheres to the foods rich in polyphenols for a drawn out timeframe, it can "trigger the sirtuin pathway to assist trigger with weighting loss". Sirtuins are specific proteins which are accepted to "shield cells in the body from biting the dust when they are under pressure and are thought to manage irritation, digestion and the maturing procedure."

Regarding tremendous research and to what extent this diet has really been near, it's still youthful and there hasn't been sufficient inside and out examination concerning the dependable impacts of keeping up a diet of just these kinds of foods for an all-encompassing timeframe.

CHAPTER 8: SIDE EFFECTS & SAFETY

Practically all medicines and medications produce undesirable reactions. Everybody is special and it is beyond the realm of imagination to expect to foresee what symptoms will happen after a SIRT methodology — a few people may have a couple of reactions while others might be progressively influenced. It is essential to talk about the potential advantages and dangers of treatment with your PCP so you will have practical desires for your treatment. The symptoms of SIRT are commonly mellow. The most well-known reactions following a SIRT strategy are:

Tiredness: This is one of the most well-known impacts and can keep going for as long as about a month and a half. If you are feeling tired it is critical to tune in to your body and get some rest. Tiredness for the most part dies down following half a month

Loss of hunger: This is one of the most widely recognized impacts and can keep going for around a month and a half

Gentle fever: This is generally observed and may keep going for as long as seven days

Stomach torment: You may feel some torment or snugness in the belly. You might be given drug for a month after the strategy to treat aggravation of the stomach and stomach ulcers

Ailment: This may keep going for one to two days. Your PCP may endorse some ant sickness tablets (enemies of emetics) to assist you with feeling good

Irritation: You may encounter some wounding or a little irregularity where the catheter went into your crotch. If this deteriorates, make certain to tell your primary care physician

Looseness of the bowels: This is generally gentle and doesn't as a rule require treatment

Uncommon to remarkable reactions

In uncommon cases, few the radioactive microspheres may accidentally arrive at different organs in the body, for example, the gallbladder, stomach, digestive system, or pancreas causing irritation or ulceration that can be inconvenient and difficult to treat. These inconveniences are uncommon, yet if they do happen they will require extra clinical treatment.

Similarly as with some other treatment choices that are utilized to expand the endurance of patients with malignant growth, SIRT can cause serious reactions that in amazingly uncommon cases can prompt passing. You will be treated by a specialist who is extraordinarily prepared in SIRT to limit the danger of these reactions from occurring.

Impact on unborn youngsters

Patients must not get SIRT treatment if they are pregnant, and must not get pregnant (or father youngsters) inside two months of getting the treatment.

It is significant that you educate your primary care physician concerning any reactions regardless of how little they may appear, particularly if you notice any exacerbating of manifestations.

As of late, you may have known about the Sirtfood Diet, the in vogue diet that guarantees you can lose as much as 7 pounds in 7 days. Established by U.K. nourishment specialists Aidan Goggins and Glen Matten, the Sirtfood Diet vows to animate the "thin quality," or the proteins under the SIRT1 quality, to balance the impacts of irritation and weight gain, just as maturing.

The Sirtfood Diet depends on the rule that specific foods initiate sirtuin, an (exceptionally disputable) protein in the body that is claimed to help manage digestion and offer cell assurance to hinder the maturing procedure. Advocates of the diet say that eating sirtuin-rich foods like green tea, kale, blueberries, salmon, and citrus natural products can give the body a consistent metabolic lift, permitting you to get in shape quick. Such foods are additionally pressed with polyphenols, which are cell reinforcements that better your skin and heart, says Brooke Alpert, RD and creator of The Diet Detox.

The Sirtfood Diet is part into two stages. The principal stage, which endures three days, expects you to limit your every day calorie admission to 1000 calories for each day by drinking three green juices and one sirtfood-rich supper every day. (You increment your feast tally from days 4 to 7 to two dinners and two green juices for each day.) The subsequent stage, the "support" stage, endures 14 days and expects you to eat three sirtuin-rich dinners and one green juice for every day.

While the guarantee of the Sirtfood diet is fascinating (Adele and Pippa Middleton are supposedly fans), and keeping in mind that limiting your calories may in truth lead you to get in shape for the time being, the inquiry remains: is this diet really healthy, or is it simply one more senseless (and possibly hazardous) diet pattern? So far as that is concerned, is it even viable in any case?

First of all: the Sirtfood diet is as a matter of fact prohibitive. In contrast to the Keto or Paleo diets, which underline having a balanced diet, the Sirtfood diet centers intensely around checking calories. It likewise expects you to remove some significant food gatherings and cut back parts to an outrageous, if just briefly. So for the primary week or thereabouts, you may be passing up lean proteins (hamburger, poultry, and vegetables). While you're despite everything permitted to eat olive oil and pecan (the two of which are wellsprings of sirtuin), the all out day by day carbohydrate content for the main week is incredibly low — under half of what the normal dynamic person needs. It additionally needs other fundamental supplements, similar to calcium and iron.

It's additionally muddled whether sirtuin can really cause weight loss in the first place. Until this point, there have been no human examinations conclusively connecting sirtuin-rich foods to weight loss. Almost certainly, drinking juices that are high in greens and low in sugar for a large portion of the day can without much of a stretch reason transient weight loss all alone: if you're getting less calories and remaining hydrated, it bodes well that you'll shed a couple of pounds. .

Kristen Smith, MS, RD, LD, a representative for the Academy of Nutrition and Dietetics, backs this up. "It is difficult to disentangle whether the quick weight loss guaranteed in the primary seven day stretch of the diet is ascribed to the significantly low-calorie diet prescribed or identified with the fat-consuming forces of sirtuin-boosting foods," she says.

Essentially, "paying little heed to the sirtuin-boosting foods, individuals will get in shape on a 1000-calorie diet," she clarifies.

Alpert concurs. "The creators state that individuals can lose as much as 7 pounds in 7 days yet I wonder the amount of this weight really remains off for longer than one month, if that long," she clarifies.

Regardless of whether you get in shape during that first week, it could be principally water weight, which implies you may restore it once you begin taking in more calories. Truth be told, you may even put on more weight: as Men's Health has recently announced, when you lose a ton of weight rapidly, your body's digestion really eases back down, because your body is attempting to compensate for its diminished calorie admission.

Likewise with any diet, the Sirtfood Diet additionally accompanies its own reactions. While it likely won't do a lot of harm for you to eat so little for the time being, if you're not used to eating so small during the day, it can cause weakness, queasiness, impeded mental center, and cerebral pains, says Smith. It can likewise prompt disagreeable solid discharges if you're not getting enough fiber. In addition, you may get terrible breath, which can be a symptom of not eating enough.

There is, in any case, one positive: If you eat a great deal of sirtfoods over a continued timeframe, you may see enhancements in heart health due to the polyphenols in the foods you're eating, Smith says. If you keep on eating sirtfoods after you end the diet and begin to eat more calories, you'll see the advantages.

The takeaway? While it is probably going to prompt momentary weight loss, the Sirtfood diet is at last so prohibitive that it's not so much supportable. What's more, if you've at any point had a dietary problem or a confounded relationship with eating before, it's ideal to stay away from it out and out, says Alpert.

"I wouldn't suggest such a low calorie consumption for anybody. Extraordinary dieting sets individuals up for horrible dietary patterns and gorging when it's finished," she includes.

All things considered, eating more sirtuin-rich foods is without a doubt useful for your health, so you can undoubtedly bring them into your diet without restricting yourself to each supper or one squeeze in turn. There's nothing amiss with eating more fish, berries, and verdant greens (particularly because these foods are stuffed with fiber and protein), and having a green squeeze that is low in sugar could be an extraordinary expansion to a previously balanced diet.

At last, you can most likely receive the rewards of the SIRT diet without making a plunge totally. Simply ensure your segments are reasonable and you're getting your calories from a wide assortment of healthy sources — no accident dieting or squeeze fasting fundamental.

CHAPTER 9: SIRTFOOD GREEN JUICE

The Sirtfood Diet green juice is a significant piece of the Sirtfood Diet. It is incorporated among the plans remembered for the Best Sirtfood Recipes page so we figured it is useful to incorporate the formula independently here. Regardless of whether you have no aim of following the diet, the juice is stuffed brimming with supplements and would be an incredible expansion to a customary diet. One significant thing to note: We have inquired about cautiously and you completely need to make this in a juicer, NOT a blender (or a Nutribullet or food processor or whatever else other than a juicer). We have given the two different ways a shot and can report that the mixed form is a frightful tasting ooze, the squeezed adaptation is a sensibly decent tasting juice!

The Sirtfood Diet green juice will keep for as long as 3 days in the refrigerator, so it's well worth making up a major cluster to spare time. We as a rule make the juices up the prior night to spare time in the mornings. This Sirtfood Diet green juice is pressed with supplements rich Sirtfoods, incredible for anybody needing somewhat of a health lift and fundamental for anybody following the Sirtfood Diet.

Fixings

- 75g kale
- 30g rocket
- 5g parsley
- 2 celery sticks
- ½ green apple
- 1cm ginger
- Juice of ½ lemon
- ½ teaspoon matcha green tea

Strategy

Squeeze all the fixings separated from the lemon and the matcha green tea.

Press the lemon juice into the green squeeze by hand.

Pour a limited quantity of green juice into a glass and mix in the matcha. Include the remainder of the green juice into the glass and mix once more.

Drink straight away or put something aside for some other time.

CHAPTER 10: RECIPES

Superfoods are probably the most healthfully thick nourishments on earth. While a considerable lot of us are simply getting on to the super food pattern, many have been utilized for a huge number of years by indigenous individuals as different types of common prescription. These force stuffed nourishments arrive in an assortment of structures from seeds, berries, gels and powders, each accompanying a different advantage.

1. Orange, Fig and Baobab Cheesecake

Recall the baobab tree from "The Little Prince?" Who might have believed that baobab was a superfoods in addition to it tastes extraordinary! This Orange, Fig and Baobab Cheesecake is a tasty, velvety treat that is made altogether of common entire nourishments so you can appreciate each significant piece!

2. Goji Berry and Hazelnut Cacao Truffles

Goji berries are little yet enthusiastic about nourishment. These Goji Berry and Hazelnut Cacao Truffles are abounded in squashed goji berries. They're brisk and simple, crude, veggie lover, sans gluten, without dairy, paleo-accommodating, no-heat, and no have no refined sugar. Gracious definitely, they're extremely scrumptious as well!

3. Mint Matcha Chip Ice Cream

This Mint Matcha Chocolate Chip Ice Cream is smooth, liberal and bravo! It has matcha green tea in it which gives it shading as well as it's a super food. In addition to the fact that this is anything but difficult to make thus reviving, it'll immediately turn into your new most loved flavor!

4. Bubbly Coconut, Lime and Mint Kombucha Elixir

This Fizzy Coconut, Lime and Mint Kombucha Elixir is reviving, tastes astonishing, looks beautiful, is hydrating, feeding and loaded with solid probiotics! Both coconut and fermented tea are considered superfoods. Check out it at home and intrigue companions with this pretty mocktail.

5. Crude Chocolate Mint Grasshopper Pie

This Raw Chocolate Mint Grasshopper Pie is a genuine group pleaser and ideal for an uncommon event with loved ones. Where's the super food? Spirulina, a sort of green growth, gives this pie its beautiful shading and huge amounts of solid supplements.

6. Rainbow Vegetable Saffron Millet Croquettes

Antiquated grains are superfoods and it's enjoyable to attempt new ones you may not be comfortable with like millet. These Rainbow Vegetable Saffron Millet Croquettes are an incredible method to attempt it. The outside gets fresh and within remains delicate. You'll begin to look all starry eyed at this grain and this dish.

7. Kimchi Kale Salad

Aged nourishments are superfoods and an extraordinary method to get probiotics into your diet. Eating kimchi, a Korean dish like sauerkraut, is a heavenly method to do it. Kimchi includes such a lot of flavor, surface, and shading to nourishment. The crunch and harshness are particularly brilliant right now Salad made with avocado, kneaded kale, chickpeas, and broiled sweet potatoes – which all happen to be superfoods too.

8. Hand crafted Dark Chocolate Chunks

Genuine chocolate – the sort accepted to hold enchanted, or even celestial, properties. All things considered, we have been hearing that a tad of dim chocolate is useful for the heart and certainly for the spirit. This Homemade Dark Chocolate Chunks formula lets you control the measure of sweetness and salt in your chocolate. That is the excellence of making your own.

9. Broiled Cauliflower and Avocado Cream Pitas

Cauliflower and avocado are both dietary powerhouses and these Roasted Cauliflower and Avocado Cream Pitas are the tastiest approach to practice good eating habits. The spiced broiled cauliflower and avocado cream are an agreeable flavor blend that preferences great on totally anything.

10. Best Ever Forbidden Rice Salad

Dark rice is a super food and the way that it's called prohibited rice just makes it much progressively captivating. This Forbidden Rice Salad is simple, fast, and ensured to intrigue. Dark rice has a simmered nutty flavor and matches well with a wide range of veggies and greens. The ginger miso dressing goes splendidly with the sweet potatoes and nutty rice.

11. Zesty Kale and Quinoa Black Bean Salad

Kale and quinoa are both superfoods. When you set up them with solid dark beans right now and Quinoa Black Bean Salad, you have a wholesome trifecta! Dark colored rice, dark beans, peppers, corn, salsa, lettuce, and guacamole – what's not to adore?

12. Chia Pudding with Blueberries

Chia seeds are sound and berries are additionally superfoods. This Chia Pudding with Blueberries is smooth, sweet and sustaining. This treat is so liberal and delectable, you'll overlook it's beneficial for you.

13. Plantain Sweet Potato Tacos with Guacamole

These Plantain Sweet Potato Tacos with Guacamole are actually as they sound – loaded down with plantains, sweet potatoes and dark beans and bested with a basic guacamole. They're veggie lover, sans gluten and a phenomenal lunch or supper alternative!

14. Chocolate Einkorn Cake

Is it cake? Is it a brownie? Whatever you call it, this Chocolate Einkorn Cake is delightful. It's a super chocolately, not excessively sweet, wet cake-brownie bar … and it's incredible. Einkorn wheat is old wheat that has never been hereditarily modified so it's solid and simpler to process.

15. Coconut Flour Porridge with Roasted Apricots

Did you realize that coconut flour makes a thick and delightful gluten and without grain porridge? Disregard your common cereal and attempt this yummy, simple breakfast of Coconut Flour Porridge! It's particularly delicious when topped with sweet caramelized apricots, however mess around with your own preferred garnishes.

16. Sound Hearty Whole Wheat Pancakes with Flax

It's constantly enjoyable to add foods grown from the ground to the hitter yet in some cases you need a flapjack formula that is somewhat more unbiased in enhance. A formula that asks for sweet fixings and a streaming waterway of maple syrup. However, obviously, it despite everything must be sound. These Healthy Hearty Whole Wheat Pancakes fit the bill impeccably. They top you off with Omega rich flax all while as yet tasting flavorful close by some new leafy foods mug of espresso or tea.

17. Spring Onion Farro Fritters With Fresh Peas, Asparagus, Radish and Tahini Mint Dressing

If farro is another grain for you, these Spring Onion Farro Fritters with Fresh Peas, Asparagus and Radishes are an extraordinary method to get presented. They are entire nourishments, plant-based thus scrumptious. Present with the mint tahini dressing which is tasty and furthermore solid.

18. Bahn Mi Salad with Pickled Vegetables and Vietnamese Croutons

Cured nourishments are superfoods and this Banh Mi Salad with Pickled Vegetables is a super dish. It's loaded up with dynamic flavors and the Vietnamese bread garnishes on top include crunch. This formula serves two huge plates of mixed greens and is veggie lover, protein-pressed and without nut with a sans gluten alternative accessible.

19. Crude Apple Pie with Goji Berries and Nutmeg

You might be thinking about how crusty fruit-filled treat can be a super food? When it's this Raw Apple Pie with Goji Berries and Nutmeg, it can. It has sound apples, super food goji berries and its crude so there's no batter. It is as nutritious as it is delectable! It is additionally exquisite topped with coconut yogurt.

20. Avocado and Veggie Spring Rolls

Avocados are superfoods and we are so cheerful about that. These Avocado and Veggie Spring Rolls are so flavorful. Loaded up with crunchy veggies and velvety avocado with bunches of Asian flavors, we prescribe making a great deal in light of the fact that these will vanish before your eyes.

21. Broccoli and Coconut Soup

This Broccoli and Coconut Soup is a lively, delightful and exceptionally nutritious mix of broccoli, spinach, lemon, ginger, and coconut milk that will warm you and feed you through the cooler winter months or just whenever you have to heat up inside.

22. Wild Rice Salad with Orange, Sweet Potato, Cherries and Pecans

This Wild Rice Salad is so pretty thus bravo. It's overflowing with a wide range of superfoods. Zest up your typical plate of mixed greens life with this delicious mix of wild rice, sweet potato, orange, fruits, and walnuts. It's the best of fall in a bowl!

23. Dark Bean Hemp Burgers

These Black Bean Hemp Burgers are so ideal for lunch, supper, nibble, even breakfast. They're likewise an ideal travel partner that will get together effectively and keep you full for a considerable length of time, on account of all the protein, fiber, and supplements.

24. Fig Hazelnut Rosemary Granola with Fig Breakfast 'Decent' Cream

Dried figs are superfoods and they're doubly solid right now Rosemary Granola with Fig Breakfast 'Decent' Cream since they are utilized twice! This yummy breakfast combo has dried figs that make the granola magnificently chewy and solidified green figs zoomed up until cushy in the "pleasant" cream.

25. Green Bean and Wild Rice Salad

When served warm, this Green Bean and Wild Rice Salad is sufficiently healthy to eat during even the coldest winter months and it has a few superfoods in it. Crunchy almonds, chewy cranberries and sun-dried tomatoes, tart olives, and generous wild rice give an intriguing blend of surfaces that will make them desire more!

Healthfully, there is nothing of the sort as a super food.

The term was instituted for showcasing purposes to impact nourishment patterns and sell items.

The nourishment business offers the super food name on supplement rich food sources with an alleged ability to decidedly influence wellbeing.

Despite the fact that numerous nourishments could be depicted as super, it's imperative to comprehend that there is no single nourishment that holds the way to great wellbeing or infection counteraction.

Be that as it may, since the expression "super food" doesn't appear to be going anyplace at any point in the near future, it might merit investigating some sound alternatives.

Here are 16 nourishments that might be deserving of the regarded super food title.

1. Dim Leafy Greens

Dim green verdant vegetables (DGLVs) are a magnificent wellspring of supplements including folate, zinc, calcium, iron, magnesium, nutrient C and fiber.

Some portion of what makes DGLVs so super is their capability to diminish your danger of ceaseless sicknesses including coronary illness and type 2 diabetes.

They likewise contain significant levels of mitigating mixes known as carotenoids, which may ensure against particular sorts of malignant growth.

Some notable DGLVs include:

- Kale
- Swiss chard
- Collard greens
- Turnip greens
- Spinach

Some DGLVs have a harsh taste and not every person appreciates them plain. You can get imaginative by remembering them for your preferred soups, servings of mixed greens, smoothies, sautés and curries.

Synopsis

Dull green verdant vegetables are brimming with fiber and supplements which might be instrumental in forestalling certain incessant illnesses.

2. Berries

Berries are a healthful powerhouse of nutrients, minerals, fiber and cell reinforcements.

The solid cell reinforcement limit of berries is related with a diminished danger of coronary illness, malignant growth and other incendiary conditions.

Berries may likewise be successful in treating different stomach related and resistant related issue when utilized close by conventional medicinal treatments.

Probably the most widely recognized berries include:

- Raspberries
- Strawberries

- Blueberries
- Blackberries
- Cranberries

Regardless of whether you appreciate them as a component of your morning meal, as a treat, on a plate of mixed greens or in a smoothie, the medical advantages of berries are as flexible as their culinary applications.

Outline

Berries are loaded with supplements and cell reinforcements which may forestall certain illnesses and improve absorption.

3. Green Tea

Initially from China, green tea is a delicately jazzed refreshment with a wide exhibit of restorative properties.

Green tea is wealthy in cancer prevention agents and polyphenolic mixes which have solid mitigating impacts. One of the most common cell reinforcements in green tea is the catechin epigallocatechin gallate, or EGCG.

EGCG is likely what gives green tea its clear capacity to ensure against ceaseless sicknesses including coronary illness, diabetes and disease.

Research likewise demonstrates that the blend of catechins and caffeine in green tea may make it a viable instrument for weight loss in certain individuals.

Rundown

Green tea is cell reinforcement rich with numerous medical advantages including conceivable malignant growth avoidance.

4. Eggs

Eggs have truly been a disputable point in the nourishment world because of their elevated cholesterol content, yet they stay perhaps the most advantageous nourishment.

Entire eggs are plentiful in numerous supplements including B nutrients, choline, selenium, nutrient an, iron and phosphorus.

They're additionally stacked with top notch protein.

Eggs contain two strong cancer prevention agents, zeaxanthin and lutein, which are known to ensure vision and eye wellbeing.

In spite of fears encompassing egg utilization and elevated cholesterol, investigate demonstrates no quantifiable increment in coronary illness or diabetes hazard from eating up to 6–12 eggs for each week.

Truth be told, eating eggs could expand "great" HDL cholesterol in certain individuals, which may prompt a good decrease in coronary illness hazard. More research is expected to reach a distinct determination.

Rundown

Eggs are wealthy in great protein and one of a kind cancer prevention agents. Research demonstrates that eating eggs normally won't expand your danger of coronary illness or diabetes.

5. Vegetables

Vegetables, or heartbeats, are a class of plant nourishments made up of beans (counting soy), lentils, peas, peanuts and horse feed.

They procure the super food mark since they're stacked with supplements and assume a job in forestalling and overseeing different maladies.

Vegetables are a rich wellspring of B nutrients, different minerals, protein and fiber.

Research shows that they offer numerous medical advantages including improved sort 2 diabetes the board, just as decreased circulatory strain and cholesterol.

Eating beans and vegetables routinely may likewise advance sound weight support, because of their capacity to improve sentiments of completion.

Outline

Vegetables are plentiful in numerous nutrients, protein and fiber. They may forestall some constant infections and bolster weight loss.

6. Nuts and Seeds

Nuts and seeds are wealthy in fiber, veggie lover protein and heart-solid fats.

They additionally pack different plant mixes with calming and cell reinforcement properties, which can secure against oxidative pressure.

Research shows that eating nuts and seeds can have a defensive impact against coronary illness.

Basic nuts and seeds include:

Almonds, walnuts, pistachios, pecans, cashews, Brazil nuts, macadamia nuts.

Peanuts — in fact a vegetable, yet often thought to be a nut.

Sunflower seeds, pumpkin seeds, chia seeds, flaxseeds, hemp seeds.

Strikingly, despite the fact that nuts and seeds are calorically thick, a few kinds of nuts are connected to weight loss when remembered for a decent diet.

Rundown

Nuts and seeds are brimming with fiber and heart-sound fats. They may lessen your danger of coronary illness and bolster weight loss.

7. Kefir (And Yogurt)

Kefir is a matured drink generally produced using milk that contains protein, calcium, B nutrients, potassium and probiotics.

Kefir is like yogurt yet has a more slender consistency and regularly more probiotic strains than yogurt.

Aged, probiotic-rich nourishments like kefir have a few related medical advantages, including decreased cholesterol, brought down pulse, improved absorption and calming impacts.

Despite the fact that kefir is generally produced using dairy animals' milk, it's ordinarily all around endured by individuals with lactose prejudice because of the maturation of the lactose by microscopic organisms.

Nonetheless, it's likewise produced using non-dairy drinks, for example, coconut milk, and rice milk and coconut water.

You can buy kefir or make it yourself. If you're picking a financially arranged item, be aware of included sugar.

Outline

Kefir is an aged dairy drink with numerous medical advantages identified with its probiotic content. In spite of the fact that by and large produced using bovine's milk, kefir is additionally accessible in non-dairy structures.

8. Garlic

Garlic is a plant nourishment that is firmly identified with onions, leeks and shallots. It's a decent wellspring of manganese, nutrient C, nutrient B6, selenium and fiber.

Garlic is a mainstream culinary fixing because of its unmistakable flavor, however it has likewise been utilized for its therapeutic advantages for a considerable length of time.

Research shows that garlic might be powerful in diminishing cholesterol and circulatory strain, just as supporting invulnerable capacity.

In addition, sulfur-containing mixes in garlic may even assume a job in forestalling specific sorts of malignant growth.

Outline

Garlic is a supplement rich nourishment utilized for its restorative advantages for a considerable length of time. It might be helpful for supporting invulnerable capacity and lessening your danger of coronary illness and certain tumors.

9. Olive Oil

Olive oil is a characteristic oil extricated from the product of olive trees and one of the pillars of the Mediterranean diet.

Its greatest cases to wellbeing are its significant levels of monounsaturated unsaturated fats (MUFAs) and polyphenolic mixes.

Adding olive oil to your diet may diminish irritation and your danger of specific ailments, for example, coronary illness and diabetes.

It additionally contains cancer prevention agents, for example, nutrients E and K, which can shield against cell harm from oxidative pressure.

Outline

Olive oil is one of the standard fat sources in the Mediterranean diet. It might be valuable in lessening coronary illness, diabetes and other provocative conditions.

10. Ginger

Ginger originates from the foundation of a blossoming plant from China. It's utilized as both a culinary flavor enhancer and for its numerous restorative impacts.

Ginger root contains cell reinforcements, for example, gingerol, that might be answerable for huge numbers of the announced medical advantages related with this nourishment.

Ginger might be successful for overseeing queasiness and lessening torment from intense and constant fiery conditions.

It might likewise lessen your danger of constant sicknesses, for example, coronary illness, dementia and certain malignant growths.

Ginger is accessible crisp, as an oil or squeeze and in dried/powdered structures. It's anything but difficult to fuse into soups, sautés, sauces and teas.

Outline

Ginger is utilized for its flavor and potential restorative impacts. It might be valuable in treating sickness, torment and forestalling certain interminable illnesses.

11. Turmeric (Curcumin)

Turmeric is a brilliant yellow flavor that is firmly identified with ginger. Initially from India, it's utilized for cooking and its restorative advantages.

Curcumin is the dynamic compound in turmeric. It has intense cancer prevention agent and mitigating impacts and is the focal point of most research encompassing turmeric.

Studies show that curcumin might be powerful in treating and forestalling constant infections, for example, malignancy, coronary illness and diabetes.

It might likewise help wound mending and agony decrease.

One downside of utilizing curcumin restoratively is that it's not effectively consumed by your body, yet its ingestion can be improved by matching it with fats or different flavors, for example, dark pepper.

Outline

The dynamic compound in turmeric, curcumin, is related with a few restorative impacts. Curcumin isn't effectively retained and ought to be combined with substances that upgrade its assimilation, for example, dark pepper.

12. Salmon

Salmon is a profoundly nutritious fish stuffed with sound fats, protein, B nutrients, potassium and selenium.

It's probably the best wellspring of omega-3 unsaturated fats, which are known for an assortment of medical advantages, for example, diminishing irritation.

Remembering salmon for your diet may likewise bring down your danger of coronary illness and diabetes and assist you with keeping up a sound weight.

A potential disadvantage of eating salmon and different kinds of fish is their conceivable tainting with substantial metals and other natural poisons.

You can stay away from potential negative impacts by restricting your utilization of fish to a few servings for every week (41).

Synopsis

Salmon is a decent wellspring of numerous supplements, particularly omega-3 unsaturated fats. Point of confinement your utilization of salmon to keep away from potential negative impacts from contaminants basic in fish and fish.

13. Avocado

Avocado is an exceptionally nutritious natural product, however it's often treated progressively like a vegetable in culinary applications.

It's plentiful in numerous supplements, including fiber, nutrients, minerals and sound fats.

Like olive oil, avocado is high in monounsaturated fats (MUFAs). Oleic corrosive is the most transcendent MUFA in avocado, which is connected to diminished irritation in the body.

Eating avocado may decrease your danger of coronary illness, diabetes, metabolic disorder and specific kinds of malignant growth.

Outline

Avocados are supplement rich, high-fiber natural products that may assume a job in diminishing irritation and ceaseless infections.

14. Sweet Potato

The sweet potato is a root vegetable stacked with numerous supplements, including potassium, fiber and nutrients An and C.

They're additionally a decent wellspring of carotenoids, a sort of cell reinforcement that may lessen your danger of specific kinds of malignant growth.

In spite of their sweet flavor, sweet potatoes don't build glucose as much as you would anticipate. Curiously, they may really improve glucose control in those with type 2 diabetes.

Outline

Sweet potatoes are a profoundly nutritious nourishment stacked with carotenoids, which have solid cell reinforcement properties. They may likewise be advantageous for glucose control.

15. Mushrooms

The absolute most regular assortments of eatable mushrooms are button, portobello, shiitake, crimini and clam mushrooms.

Despite the fact that supplement content changes relying upon the sort, mushrooms contain nutrient A, potassium, fiber, and a few cell reinforcements not present in most different nourishments.

Strikingly, eating more mushrooms is related with more noteworthy utilization of vegetables all in all, adding to a general progressively nutritious diet.

Because of their one of a kind cell reinforcement content, mushrooms may likewise assume a job in lessening irritation and forestalling specific sorts of malignancies.

Another super element of mushrooms is that rural waste items are utilized to develop them. This makes mushrooms a supportable part of a sound nourishment framework.

Outline

Mushrooms are loaded with supplements and may decrease your danger of specific ailments. Furthermore, mushrooms are a manageable nourishment decision.

16. Kelp

Kelp is a term used to portray certain supplement rich ocean vegetables. It's most normally devoured in Asian food however is picking up notoriety in different pieces of the world because of its healthy benefit.

Ocean growth packs numerous supplements, including nutrient K, folate, iodine and fiber.

These sea vegetables are a wellspring of novel bioactive mixes — not ordinarily show in land-vegetables — which may have cell reinforcement impacts.

A portion of these mixes may likewise diminish your danger of malignant growth, coronary illness, heftiness and diabetes.

Synopsis

Ocean growth is a gathering of exceptionally nutritious ocean vegetables that may assume a job in ensuring against certain interminable illnesses.

1. Greek Yogurt

Regular yogurt's thicker, creamier cousin is crammed with protein and probiotics. It fills the gut, improves absorption, and reinforces the insusceptible framework. Furthermore, it's an extraordinary sound formula substitute for sharp cream, cream cheddar, and even mayonnaise!

2. Quinoa

This minuscule, grain-like seed packs some genuine dietary ability. With a mellow, nutty flavor and a surface like rice or couscous, quinoa is one of the main grains or seeds that gives every one of the nine basic amino acids our bodies can't deliver themselves. Also, it's loaded up with protein—eight grams for each one-cup serving, to be careful!

3. Blueberries

Don't stress; these berries won't cause an oompa-loompa-like response. Actually, they're wholesome geniuses, loaded up with fiber, nutrient C, and malignancy battling mixes. Furthermore, considers propose blueberries may even improve memory!

4. Kale

This unpleasant and intense green prevails over all the rest regarding sustenance, giving a greater number of cancer prevention agents than most different foods grown from the ground! It's likewise a phenomenal wellspring of fiber, calcium, and iron. Set it up basically any way, from bubbled or steamed to broiled (attempt it as a chip!) or stewed.

5. Chia

Ch-ch-ch-chia! That's right, this little seed is equivalent to those delightful minimal artistic creature grower of the 90s! In any case, don't stress, the nutritious part isn't the dirt pot. Chia seeds are really stacked with the most basic unsaturated fats of any known plant! Additionally, one serving of the stuff is stacked with magnesium, iron, calcium, and potassium.

6. Cereal

High in fiber, cell reinforcements, and huge amounts of different supplements, this morning meal staple has been appeared to help lower cholesterol levels, help in processing, and even improve digestion. What's more, it's out and out scrumptious—particularly when seasoned like pumpkin pie!

7. Green Tea

This ages-old wellbeing mystery has been utilized as a characteristic solution for everything from malignant growth to coronary illness! The key to this heavenly drink? Cell reinforcements! The fundamental hero here is Epigallocatechin gallate, or EGCG, a phytochemical that eases back unpredictable cell development, which might help forestall the development of certain malignancies.

8. Broccoli

This lean, mean, green machine is pressed with nutrients, minerals, ailment battling mixes, and the fiber basic in any diet. In spite of the fact that all individuals from the cruciferous vegetable family are super sound, broccoli stands apart for its outstandingly elevated levels of nutrient C and folate (which can diminish danger of coronary illness, certain tumors, and stroke).

9.Strawberries

Vitamin C is the genius of this super food. Only one cup of these red wonders fulfills the everyday necessity for nutrient C (74 milligrams for each day for ladies, 90 for men)! Studies propose the cell reinforcement helps fabricate and fix the body's tissues, supports insusceptibility, and battles overabundance free extreme harm. What's more, the nutrient C in strawberries could help advance solid eye work.

10. Salmon

This heart-solid fish is pressed with protein and a sound portion of omega-3 unsaturated fats, which studies recommend may help diminish the danger of cardiovascular illness. What's more, extra focuses: Salmon may likewise shield skin from the sun and the harming impacts of UV beams.

11. Watermelon

Low in sugar and high in nutrients An and C, this midyear treat is the ideal, amazing failure calorie nibble. Studies recommend watermelon could likewise possibly bring down circulatory strain and diminish the danger of cardiovascular sickness. Furthermore, the lycopene in watermelon could help shield the body from UV beams and malignant growth.

12. Spinach

Antioxidants, hostile to inflammatory, and nutrients that advance vision and bone wellbeing are what make this green so super. What's more, those bones will thank spinach, as well! Only one cup of the stuff gets together to 12 percent of the suggested day by day portion of calcium and enough nutrient K to help forestall bone loss.

13. Pistachios

These lil' nuts are concealing loads of protein and fiber behind their hearty flavor and nutty crunch. In addition, they're normally sans cholesterol. A one-ounce serving of these nuts has nearly as a lot of potassium as one little banana.

14. Eggs

A moderately cheap protein source stacked with supplements, eggs positively acquire their super food status. A solitary huge egg is just around 70 calories and offers six grams of protein. Eggs are likewise an extraordinary wellspring of omega-3 unsaturated fats, which are fundamental for ordinary body capacity and heart wellbeing.

15. Almonds

Surprise! Almonds are the most healthfully thick nut, which means they offer the most elevated centralization of supplements per calorie per ounce. For only 191 calories, a one-ounce serving gives 3.4 grams of fiber (that is around 14 percent of the everyday suggested esteem) and a solid portion of potassium, calcium, nutrient E, magnesium, and iron. Furthermore, you can eat them as BUTTER!

16. Ginger

Slightly zesty yet quite pleasant, ginger has been utilized for quite a long time as a delectable enhancing and an all-characteristic solution for everything from a steamed stomach to undesirable irritation.

17. Beets

This elite player veggie contains huge amounts of nutrients, minerals, and cell reinforcements that can help battle ailment and strengthen indispensable organs. Also, their purple tint might be the key to their sound achievement—a few examinations recommend betalains, the purple shades in these veggies, may assist ward with offing malignant growth and other degenerative sicknesses.

18. Beans

High in protein and low in cholesterol, beans of any assortment can add a sound wind to any dish (even brownies!). They're likewise stacked with fiber, folate, and magnesium, and studies have demonstrated that vegetables (like beans) can really help lower cholesterol and decrease the danger of specific diseases (at any rate in rodents).

19. Pumpkin

Loaded with cancer prevention agents and nutrients, these gourds aren't only for cutting (or making into pie). The star supplement here is beta-carotene, a provitamin that the body changes over to nutrient A, which is known for its resistant boosting forces and fundamental job in eye wellbeing.

20. Apples

Say it with us, individuals: "Fiber is acceptable." And apples are an incredible low-calorie source. (A medium-sized apple tips the scales at under 100 calories.) Plus, increasing apple consumption has been related with decreased danger of cardiovascular sickness, certain malignant growths, diabetes, and asthma.

21. Cranberries

It's an ideal opportunity to work these fall top choices into dishes all year. Regardless of whether it's looking like a can or new off the stove, cranberries have a bunch of medical advantages and illness battling powers. These microscopic organisms busting berries can help battle irritation, lessen the danger of coronary illness, improve oral wellbeing, help forestall ulcers and yeast contaminations, and may even restrain the development of some human malignant growth cells.

22. Garlic

Yes, it may leave breath not exactly attractive, yet these cloves can accomplish more than season—they've been utilized for a considerable length of time as nourishment and drug. Nowadays, garlic is utilized to treat anything from hypertension and coronary illness to specific kinds of malignant growth. Also, considers recommend garlic concentrate can be utilized to treat yeast diseases in ladies and prostate issues in men.

23. Cauliflower

While every one of the nutrients and minerals are an extraordinary reward, the genuine star here is cauliflower's disease battling mixes, glucosinolates. These phytochemicals are answerable for cauliflower's occasionally harsh flavor, yet they have additionally been appeared to forestall harm to the lungs and stomach via cancer-causing agents, possibly ensuring against those malignant growths. Furthermore, on account of communications with estrogen, cauliflower may likewise help forestall hormone-driven malignant growths like bosom, uterine, and cervical.

The makers of the sirtfood diet guarantee that by eating these foods, you actuate your "thin quality," and this can reflect the impacts of fasting and exercise. Among the food things: arugula, buckwheat, tricks, cocoa, espresso, green tea, kale, Medjool dates, red wine, strawberries and turmeric.

Dieters focus on two stages and a three-week time-range:

Stage 1: Consume 1,000 calories day by day for three days, comprising of three sirtfood green juices (see formula further down) and one sirtfood-rich feast (if you need inspo, the diet's designers share sirtfood plans on their site). For the rest of the week, calorie consumption ascends to 1,500 calories every day with two green juices and two suppers.

Stage 2: Meal plan involves three sirtfood-stuffed suppers, two or three tidbits and one sirtfood green juice for every day for the following 14 days.

Then, keep up the diet by ceaselessly eating foods rich in sirtuins at each supper and drinking that mark green juice.

(Additionally, note the diet, as most, supports standard exercise too.)

Sirtfood Green Juice Recipe

(Serves 1)

- Machine
- One juicer
- Fixings
- 2 huge bunches (2.5 oz) kale
- a huge bunch (1 oz) arugula
- small bunch (1/4 oz) level leaf parsley

- 2 to 3 huge (5.5 oz) celery stems, including leaves
- ½ medium green apple
- ½-to 1-inch piece new ginger
- juice of ½ lemon
- ½ level teaspoon matcha powder

Bearings: Mix kale, arugula and parsley together, then squeeze them. Next, juice celery, apple and ginger. Press lemon by hand into the juice. Empty a touch of juice into a glass, include matcha, mix and hang tight for it to disintegrate. Include rest of juice, include a last mix, drink or top with plain water.

Masters and Cons of the Sirtfood Diet

Per the makers, health advantages of this "diet of consideration" incorporate improved memory work, held bulk, better controlled glucose levels and diminished danger of ceaseless illness. A pilot test discovered members lost a normal seven pounds in seven days while keeping up or expanding bulk and saw better vitality, rest and skin improvement.

In any case, for all said favorable circumstances, the diet isn't without its doubters. A USA Today book proposes "the science isn't there in people to help a portion of their cases that it initiates the 'thin quality' and can support digestion and increment fat-consuming." The International Food Information Council echoes that idea, expressing the sirtfood diet is "not science-based or feasible."

What's more, to the extent that pilot study goes? The outcomes are "not really astonishing," says a Healthline post. "Limiting your calorie admission to 1,000 calories and practicing simultaneously will almost consistently cause weight loss"... noticing, "This investigation didn't follow members after the primary week" to check whether weight gain returned.

The concept of sirtfoods

Genuine talk, when I initially read about this diet, I thought it was made up. Sirtfood? What the hell is that – spell check is demanding it's not so much as a word. Be that as it may, as most things in our insane diet industry, it's not made up, thus called specialists are considering it the enchantment projectile of weight loss. In this post, we'll see whether this diet is the most important thing in the world everything being equal and what proof exists to back that up.

I gotta concede, most of the time, you'll see me on the Adele train. I'm the first to wrench up her tunes and dream about the day we are at last rejoined as tragically deceased sisters, however my reality came smashing down when she uncovered her weight loss counteractant The Sirtfood diet. Honestly, I boycotted her music for one day. I could just deal with one day because we should be genuine... it's Adele. Rather than taking out the entirety of my dissatisfaction on an artist with most likely almost no nourishment skill, I chose we'd discover who was defiling her with this data and carry them and their examination to equity.

The Sirtfood diet was created by two nourishment scientists that as of late co-composed a book about the diet. Before you run out and get it, we should set aside you some cash and give you the abject here.

The Sirtfood diet underscores eating foods that may connect with a group of proteins known as sirtuin proteins (presently the name of the diet is beginning to bode well). Sirtuins have been intensely examined and primer examinations have indicated some encouraging advantages. Every individual from the sirtuin family assumes an indispensable job in directing things like our digestion, interior body clock, life span and maturing. Because of the job they play in digestion, a few specialists are calling sirtuins "thin qualities" for their potential job in weight loss.

Adele's emotional weight loss has had the web totally fixated. She originally appeared a slimmer constitution in October a year ago, however in the wake of showing up at Beyonce and Jay-Z's Oscars after-party having allegedly lost a stunning 99 pounds (45kgs), it's everything anybody can discuss. Everybody is kicking the bucket to realize what her mystery is.

The appropriate response? The Sirtfood Diet.

This "inexplicable" and "game-changing" diet claims you'll lose a normal of 6.5 pounds (3kgs) in the primary week.

Peruse on to discover all that you have to think about the Sirtfood Diet and whether it'll work for you.

In light of research on sirtuins (SIRTs), SIRTs are a gathering of seven proteins found in the body that has appeared to direct an assortment of capacities. These incorporate digestion, irritation, and lifespan. "Sirtfoods" are foods high in sirtuin activators.

The Sirtfood Diet works by consolidating "sirtfoods" and calorie limitation. The two of which work to trigger the body to deliver more elevated levels of sirtuins.

How does the Sirtfood Diet work?

The Sirtfood Diet has a rebuffing notoriety. It works in two stages. Stage one sees adherents constrained to a measly 1000 calories every day for the initial three days. These calories comprise of three green smoothies and one little dinner.

Between days four to seven, the calorie consumption ascends to 1,500, comprised of two green smoothies and two little sirtfood-rich dinners.

Then, Phase Two, which goes on for about fourteen days and spotlights on support.

There is no specified calorie admission for this period. Despite the fact that you're required to eat three suppers of sirtfood-rich foods and one green juice for each day, you'll keep on getting more fit during this stage.

Is it economical?

Organizers of the Sirtfood Diet make strong cases. They state that the diet can super-charge weight loss, turn on your "thin quality" and forestall infections. They guarantee you'll lose a normal of 3kg every WEEK.

However, there isn't a lot of verification to back them.

Up until this point, there's no ACTUAL scientific proof that the Sirtfood Diet has a more gainful impact on weight loss than some other calorie-limited diet.

Doubtlessly that you'll shed pounds on the Sirtfood Diet. If you confined your calorie admission to 1000 and ate just chocolate, you'd STILL get more fit.

Significantly limiting calories and practicing simultaneously will quite often bring about weight loss.

If you're searching for a convenient solution weight loss arrangement that will make them drop the pounds

FAST, then sure, give the Sirtfood Diet a go. Be that as it may, at what cost?

After the two stages are finished, what then?

The Sirtfood Diet has serious limitations. The calorie necessities don't consider sexual orientation, body synthesis, and physical action level. This implies a portion of the individuals who tail it could be under eating. Under eating can make the roll over eat the next week, making you recover the weight that was lost in stage one.

If you choose to follow stage two for longer than the suggested time span and you're under eating, it can cause "metabolic adjustment", the easing back of your digestion, prompting a bounce back impact. This can bring about the individual not just recovering all the weight that they lost however conceivably putting on MORE than they began with.

Is it worth sacrificing a portion of life's most prominent delights? Delights like eating out with a friend or family member, lunch with companions, or mixed drinks with the young ladies. All because it's difficult to track down foods that not exclusively should originated from a specified rundown yet in addition fall inside an absurdly low calorie recompense?

Would it be a good idea for you to attempt the Sirtfood Diet?

With all diet prevailing fashions, they often present an alluring picture that appears to be unrealistic. The thing is, if it SEEMS unrealistic, it presumably is.

I can't resist the urge to think about how Adele will be looking, yet more critically, FEELING, a couple of years down the track. What are the drawn out ramifications of following such a tight, prohibitive diet? It's too early to realize the drawn out reactions of denying your assortment of much-required macronutrients for such an all-inclusive period.

If you're searching for long haul, feasible weight loss, then it's everything about balance.

It's tied in with discovering approaches to eat the foods you cherish and make the most of life's shared minutes without feeling confined or denied.

Including more "sirtfoods" to your diet won't hurt you, yet if you're searching for a weight-loss plan that will be pleasant and simple to follow, avoid this prevailing fashion diet.

If you're searching for a healthy, reasonable and balanced approach to assume responsibility for your weight loss venture, while eating the foods you love, IIFYM have the arrangement.

Complete with supper plans and exercise programs, altered to your accurate one of a kind needs, you'll have the opportunity to eat anything you desire as long as it accommodates your macros.

Indeed, in all honesty, you aren't even really devouring sirtuins on this diet. You're devouring foods rich in polyphenols (convey cancer prevention agent properties) that as far as anyone knows enact sirtuins.

Here's a rundown of sirtuin activator foods:

- Kale
- Dim chocolate
- Apples
- Red wine
- Citrus organic product
- Espresso

- Escapades
- Blueberries
- Parsley
- Green tea
- Soy
- Strawberries
- Turmeric
- Olive Oil
- Rocket
- Red Onion

Is the Sirtfood diet the way to weight loss over the long haul? We audit the exploration behind the now famous Sirtfood diet alongside diet claims and research on whether it works for weight loss.

The majority of the foods that have made this a feature commendable diet are wine and dim chocolate, clearly. These foods do have a spot in our diet, because their high cell reinforcement levels may help shield us from certain ceaseless illnesses and malignancies. For more data on cell reinforcements, click here to peruse my post. In any case, weight loss?

The Sirtfood diet site mentions that their diet is centered more around health as opposed to weight loss yet I call that bull s**t because the front of their diet book states: "Shed 7 pounds in 7 days".

In the book, they give you a bit by bit manage on following the diet. Here are the two stages:

SIRTFOOD DIET PHASE 1

DAY 1 – 3

During the initial three days, calories are limited to just 1000 kcal/day and every day you should expend a sirtfood green juice which contains either green tea, lovage herb as well as buckwheat. Your suppers must contain foods rich in sirtfood activators.

DAY 4 – 7

After the initial three days, your calories are expanded to 1500 kcal/day and you should expend two juices and two ordinary dinners daily.

SIRTFOOD DIET PHASE 2

DAY 8 – 22

The following fourteen days are viewed as a support period where you can eat three balanced dinners rich in sirtfood activators in addition to a green juice.

After that it's up to you whether you need to re-start the stages. This is the place the dietary proposals appeared to get unclear because they don't give a specific course of events on what number of more occasions you ought to rehash these stages. The absence of direction here makes me anxious, because tedious caloric limitation may have some drawn out suggestions which we'll talk about in a piece.

So after a progression of angry scenes and drinking heaps of green s**t, what would we be able to anticipate?

SIRTFOOD DIET CLAIMS

Is the Sirtfood diet the way to weight loss over the long haul? We survey the examination behind the now mainstream Sirtfood diet alongside diet claims and research on whether it works for weight loss.

The greatest case this diet gloats about is that these sirtuin proteins will expand our body's capacity to consume fat, advance muscle development, support and fix and as referenced before fast weight loss. Because quick weight loss is consistently protected, right?! (Embed enormous eye roll). Other non-weight related advantages include: improving memory, controlling glucose levels and shielding you from malignant growths and ceaseless ailments.

So what's the inside scoop on these thin qualities?

Proof FOR THE SIRTFOOD DIET?

Is the Sirtfood diet the way to weight loss over the long haul? We survey the examination behind the now famous Sirtfood diet alongside diet claims and research on whether it works for weight loss.

Most of studies taking a gander at the impacts of sirtuins and weight loss have just been done on rodents, yeast, worms and human foundational microorganisms. A few mice and yeast examines have indicated that a cell reinforcement known as resveratrol, found in grapes and blueberries, which enact sirtuins may imitate the activities of caloric limitation which thusly will prompt weight loss. Different investigations have discovered that resveratrol may assume a job in malignant growth counteraction, coronary illness and diabetes in creatures, however there's insufficient proof to comprehend its job in people. Something else to bring up is that a significant number of the investigations utilized are taking a gander at the segregated type of sirtuins and not sirtuins found in the food itself which separations us considerably more from solid proof. They likewise will in general utilize high portions of cell reinforcements which are unthinkable for us to try and accomplish from food sources (more wine doesn't approach more noteworthy advantages... sorry to be the unwanted messenger).

Is the Sirtfood diet the way to weight loss over the long haul? We survey the examination behind the now mainstream Sirtfood diet alongside diet claims and research on whether it works for weight loss.

The main human proof around the viability of a Sirtfood diet on weight loss originates from one clinical preliminary. This preliminary was remembered for the Sirtfood Diet book and planned by the authors themselves. Unfortunately, the clinical preliminary conveyed a great deal of powerless stuff. The pilot study had 40 members in a private exercise center in Chelsea, London. Over a 7-day time span, 39 members shed 7 pounds and their bulk was either kept up or expanded.

I can't in great cognizant stop there. Here are the plenteous constraints from this examination:

SMALL SAMPLE SIZE

Is the Sirtfood diet the way to weight loss over the long haul? We audit the exploration behind the now well known Sirtfood diet alongside diet claims and research on whether it works for weight loss.

Pilot reads are famous for being little, subsequently the term pilot study, yet at the same time we can't unquestionably suggest this diet dependent on the effect it had on 39 exercise center rabbits. A pilot study is the first of numerous examinations that ought to be led on a specific theme, and ought to not the slightest bit be the main wellspring of proof for putting forth the defense for a diet.

TEST BIAS

Is the Sirtfood diet the way to weight loss over the long haul? We audit the examination behind the now well known Sirtfood diet alongside diet claims and research on whether it works for weight loss.

The main members in the investigation were no-nonsense rec center goers who are no doubt a health cognizant populace that follow a healthy diet and exercise consistently. To state this populace is a reasonable portrayal of the remainder of humankind is a long way from the real world.

NO FOLLOW UP

Is the Sirtfood diet the way to weight loss over the long haul? We audit the exploration behind the now famous Sirtfood diet alongside diet claims and research on whether it works for weight loss.

A key estimation to test the adequacy of an intercession is to plan a development. That way you can find the members and see whether there are any drawn out advantages. Rather, they just estimated the members for seven days and that was that. This doesn't reveal to us much and whether the diet really works.

NO CONTROL GROUP

Is the Sirtfood diet the way to weight loss over the long haul? We survey the examination behind the now well-known Sirtfood diet alongside diet claims and research on whether it works for weight loss.

I have a great deal of issue with this impediment. The pith of a clinical preliminary is a benchmark group. Without one, you can't state for certain whether the mediation, for this situation the sirtfood activators, directly affected the investigation results. Sounds like total scholastic turmoil!

These constraints make for a frail report and it is by all accounts the main examination these organizers are sticking on to. So's a major warning.

Here's my concern with this diet. Beside resveratrol, something else that may actuate sirtuins is limiting calories which is the reason it's a piece of stage 1 of the diet.

CALORIE RESTRICTION

Is the Sirtfood diet the way to weight loss over the long haul? We audit the examination behind the now well-known Sirtfood diet alongside diet claims and research on whether it works for weight loss.

On numerous occasions, I've called attention to you folks the issue with most diets: prohibitive eating. When it comes to limitation, our dissident impulses need to take advantage of the man and gorge like there's no tomorrow. I'm almost certain you'll additionally turn into that companion that nobody needs to go out with because of your new angry character. Yet, for realties, there have not been sufficient reliable examinations that state calorie limitation is the best approach. Without a doubt, you'll lose some sweet poundage briefly however you'll additionally meet some unwanted results and in the long run recapture the weight. Studies taking a gander at caloric limitation found that after some time limitation prompts loss of bulk (which thoroughly counters what the sirtfood diet claims it can do), muscle quality and loss of bone, weakness, crabbiness and gloom.

CONCLUSION

If you like sirtfood activators, feel free to devour them. I have no issue with advancing an assortment of plant-based foods wealthy in health securing blessed messengers. Hell, I love a glass of red wine toward the finish of a bustling week and I can never disapprove of a bit of dull chocolate. A decent dependable guideline isn't to confide in diets that boast about shedding 7 pounds in 7 days. Most importantly, it's generally ridiculous and bogus promoting, and second of all, most of the time it's hazardous. Not at all like Adele, the vast majority of us don't approach extravagant mentors and additionally the ideal opportunity for two-a-day exercise center meetings. Until further notice, we can unquestionably say that the examination doesn't support the utilization of sirtuins for weight loss. Until further notice, in any event.